ROOM TO ROAM

More Tales of a Montana Veterinarian

BY R. W. "Rib" Gustafson, D.V.M.

Library of Congress Catalog Card Number: 96-94534

ISBN: 1-56044-497-5

Published by R. W. Gustafson, Route 1, Box 136,
Conrad, Montana 59425,
in cooperation with SkyHouse Publishers,
an imprint of Falcon Press Publishing Co., Inc.,
Helena, Montana.

Design, typesetting, and other prepress work
by Falcon Press.

Cover painting by Pat Gustafson.

Distributed by Falcon Press Publishing Co., Inc.,
P.O. Box 1718, Helena, Montana 59624,
phone 1-800-582-2665.

First Edition

Manufactured in the United States of America.

Dedicated to my wife and great family

CONTENTS

FOREWORD

When I was 12 years old, Dad had me behind the wheel of his '72 Chevy Impala perched on top of his medicine kit so I could see over the dashboard as we wound our way through the endless maze of gravel roads on the benchlands of the great Rocky Mountain Front. A trail of dust betrayed our presence and brought a welcoming smile to an old farmer anxiously awaiting our arrival. It was a great excuse for me to get out of school and learn about some of the more important things in life! Old Mother Nature and Dad were the best set of instructors a 12-year-old kid could have. The "3 R's" would be dealt with sooner or later, but nothing compared to the experience of watching a breached calf being introduced to a brisk March morning in God's country. "C-Section," "prolapse," "blackleg," "brucellosis," "pink eye," "colic" . . . weird and wonderful words that heralded my introduction to the dramatic domain of a prairie veterinarian. Words that wove their way in and out of crackling conversations on a high-powered two-way radio that was often our only link to civilization.

And the people we would meet on our journeys! Good folks with hardy northern names . . . Woldstad, McGillis, Johnson, and Rumney. Names that were synonymous with a stand of buildings or a set of corrals that marked our destination. Families that were haphazardly scattered over the endless countryside, clinging to a way of life that revolved around hard work, the will of God, and a good vet. Colorful characters in a giant play that unfolded day after day on the wide open plains of Montana. A plot that kept repeating itself with a simple choice of outcomes . . . sickness or health, life or death.

I'll never forget the joy and wonderment of watching a young cow, after inheriting a big incision and a half a box of hog rings on her underbelly, stand up and lick her calf like nothing ever happened . . . or the horror of walking into the aftermath of a covey of broomtails that breakfasted on an old sack of gopher poison. The dramas were never ending. The memories flow like the crystal-clear waters of the eastern slope. Thanks, Dad, for sharing them with us.

— Wylie Gustafson
[of Wylie and the Wild West Show]

vii

THE COWBOY'S LULLABY

He rode the night herd for the old Cross Three.
The stars up above and a pony beneath.
Through the restless bunches he'd gently parade
And sing to them softly his sweet serenade.

CHORUS:
(Yodel)
Good night little doggies, good night.
He'd bed 'em all down with the melancholy sound
Of the Cowboy's Lullaby.

He said, hush ya little dogies, I'll do ya no wrong.
Come the mornin' sun we'll be movin' on.
So sleep while ya can, dream all your dreams
Of water a plenty and great pastures of green.

CHORUS

He'd coo and he'd call till he put 'em to rest
Of all the night riders, he was the best.
Makin' the rounds from dusk until dawn,
With a jingle and a jangle he'd sing 'em his song.

CHORUS

That lonesome old cowboy don't ride anymore.
He drifted away to a far distant shore.
But if you listen closely by the prairie's full moon,
You'll hear the wind whisper his heavenly tune.

CHORUS

Words & Music by Wylie Gustafson
© TWO MEDICINE MUSIC

PREFACE

I must have been shot in the rear end with luck when I was born. I'm so lucky that my long life reaches from practically the horse-and-buggy days to today's space-age world of computers, advanced medicine, and other facets of science and our modern environment that touch us everyday.

I started the first grade sitting on an apple box way up high in the Crazy Woman Mountains in central Montana. The next year the teacher, my older brother, and I drove five miles to school in a horse and buggy to a country schoolhouse where we were met by two other children coming from the opposite direction. I even slept with the schoolteacher once——when we were snowbound in that little one-room schoolhouse for three days. It felt pretty good to cuddle up to a warm female with a raging blizzard rattling the windows and north winds drifting snow outside.

That spring, when I was seven years old, my dad died from Rocky Mountain spotted fever, leaving my mother with eight children to care for and rear. I still can remember vividly two trips to the small town of Ryegate, where we kids were inoculated against the tick-borne illness our dad caught. They shot a horse-serum vaccine into our left arms, which practically immobilized them for two days. The Rocky Mountain Laboratory in Hamilton, Montana, had recently developed the new vaccine program. Today, with our broad-spectrum antibiotics and advanced knowledge, this once-deadly disease carried around by the tick *Dermacenter andersoniae* is quite controllable.

After my father's death, and because of the severe depression that affected the whole country, we lost the ranch and all of our mortgaged livestock. Mother and kids moved into the small town of Rapelje. Since in those days there was no welfare system as there is today, my mother took in boarders to hold the family together. My older brothers found work rounding up horses and shipping them to Minnesota, where they were purchased by farmers too broke to buy the new machinery that was just beginning to replace traditional horsepower. Three of my older siblings took the money from these horse sales and entered the University of Minnesota, upon the insistence of our mother, and began the long road to higher education.

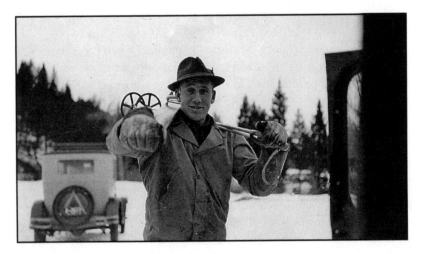

Home from the seven seas and ready to practice, 1945.

The rest of the family then moved to Bozeman, Montana, where my mother continued to take in boarders and to raise and school us younger children. I finished high school in Bozeman in 1942, enlisted in the U.S. Navy Air Corps, and returned from World War II in 1945. After much thought about continuing my career as a naval aviator, I decided I would become a veterinarian instead. With the help of the G.I. Bill, which helped defray expenses, I went on to continue my education and fulfill my life dreams.

I have now practiced veterinary medicine for more than four decades and am grateful that two of my sons have followed in the same intriguing profession. There isn't a passing day in this work that doesn't offer new challenges and enjoyable experiences. Veterinary medicine also has a vibrant past. I can't verify this, but it has been said that Napoleon failed to conquer Europe and Russia because of foot-and-mouth disease epidemics that destroyed animals by the thousands. (I'm not talking about the foot-IN-mouth disease that afflicts our politicians of today, but I sometimes wonder if that won't destroy us, too.) The virus affected the mobility of farm animals, and left starving armies to flounder. Glanders in horses put soldiers afoot and was probably the reason that oxen instead of draft horse teams pulled the wagon trains to Oregon and California during the great western migration. Blackleg and anthrax probably exterminated more buffalo on the Great Plains than did Indians and whites. Smallpox killed more Indians than wars did. If Captain Meriwether Lewis had implicitly followed President Thomas Jefferson's orders, he would have vaccinated all of the native people with whom he came in contact with "the pox of the kine"—cattle-based vaccine, which is still the vaccine in use today. Edward Jenner's observation of beautiful French milkmaids who were protected from smallpox because of the cross-immunization capabilities of "cow pox," marked a great advancement in the annals of medicine. In just the last few years, the descendant versions of his vaccine finally have freed the world from the ravages of smallpox.

There are many other instances where animals and animal doctors influenced the course of human history. Horse hair was one of the early surgical suture materials, until it was discovered that it carried the spores of anthrax. Catgut, which mainly comes from the intestinal lining of sheep, is still used extensively today. Artificial insemination, which was long used by Arabs to improve horse breeds, is another example—today we have embryo implants and alternative procedures in humans that were first developed in animals. Animal use for advancements in human medicine has been common for years, and it recently has led to moral questions involving animal rights.

Regardless of the debate, I entered what seemed to me like a noble profession. Veterinarians were scarce when I arrived in Montana's Golden Triangle in 1951 to start a practice. There had been only two bona fide practitioners here ahead of me, plus a few wannabes who people called in dire circumstances. No one was available in the rural areas for work on small companion animals or ranch dogs. They were usually taken to Great Falls, Montana, ninety miles distant, or not treated at all.

The first question asked when I arrived was, "How are you going to make a living, Rib, when others have failed?" I nearly didn't. But cattle prices were at a cyclical high. I knew folks in the region, since I had worked in the area the previous summer, operating the Shelby Stockyards for my brother Duke and his partner Danny O'Niel. (Being young and single, I had even managed to meet a few members of the opposite sex.) So I eked out a living, though it was a bad year weatherwise. Rural roads looked like snow tunnels. Since I liked to ski, I spent time traveling to the Big Mountain near Whitefish and what was then called King's Hill (now Showdown) in the Belt Mountains. At one time that winter I only had about ten dollars left to my name.

That's when the spring chinook set in, and I had one of the most delicious springtimes of my life. I had been cooped up in educational facilities for so many years that it seemed as though I'd found new freedom in the beautiful Northern Rockies. This land put a half-strangle on me that I've never wanted—or been able—to escape. In this large area, there isn't a road I haven't traveled and a permanent occupant I haven't known. The years have slipped by, and my roots have grown deeper.

I wouldn't change anything in my life—as I say, I've been lucky. Physically active, I'm still an advocate of beefsteak, bacon and eggs, immoral fantasies, and the other things that make life pleasurable—like Carl Sandburg's favorite poem of the "preacher who looked so God-damned glum when he spoke of kingdom come." Irreverence fits into my philosophy at times.

I learned in school that cancer is caused by age, environment, and heredity. I've interpolated that to mean that if we all live long enough, we will all die of cancer. I have quit smoking and drinking, so maybe that will entitle me to be warbled to by some self-appointed do-gooder in a nursing home someday. Until then, I'll enjoy life and continue to record it as I have for the many years I've spent in this Big Sky Country, where there's plenty of room to roam.

ACKNOWLEDGMENTS

I give thanks to my family and especially to son Wylie for the foreword. To my editor, Noelle Sullivan, for making it into publishing form; to Falcon Press for encouragement and distribution; to my wife, Pat, for the cover; and to all my clients who have employed me over the years. To my four sons and daughter for advice and proofreading, and to the omnipotent for the room to roam. Also, to Kim Solven for interpreting my hand writing.

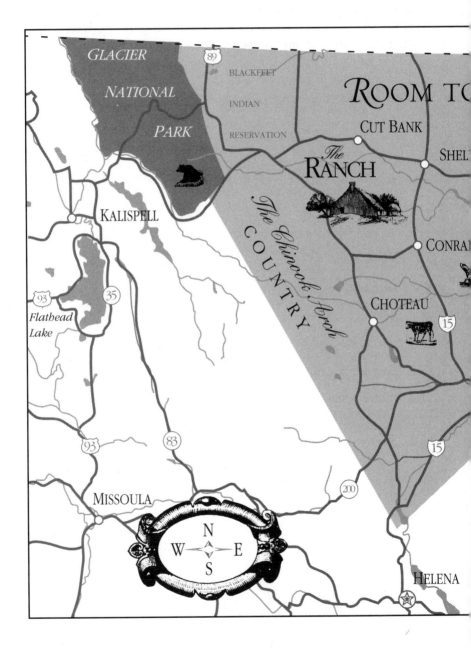

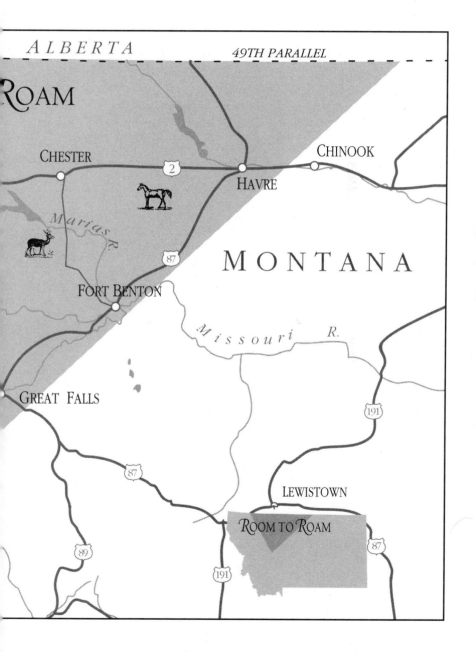

ALBERTA   *49TH PARALLEL*

ROAM

CHESTER   2   CHINOOK

HAVRE

Marias R.

87

FORT BENTON

MONTANA

Missouri R.

GREAT FALLS

191

87

LEWISTOWN

ROOM TO ROAM

89

191

87

ROOM TO ROAM

PREGNANCY DIAGNOSIS

IF A RANCHER HAS A MILLION BUCKS, he will spend it—and sometimes it doesn't take long. For every cow he owns he has close to three thousand dollars invested. For every man he hires, he has a few million dollars stuck into the business. So every fall after his calves are sold, a ranch man gets serious and wants to know how many calves he can tell his friendly banker he expects so he can borrow enough to maintain his lifestyle for another year. Efficient production of more calves is the name of the game.

That's where veterinarians come in. Pregnancy testing of a bovine involves rectal palpation, seeking sign of a fetus or development of fetal membranes in the uterus. The cow is caught in a chute and the veterinarian attacks her from the rear wearing a plastic sleeve or long rubber glove. Once the vet determines that the bull has done his job, the cow is wormed, ear-tagged, treated for external and internal parasites, and released.

Many times I have done four or five hundred pregnancy tests in an afternoon. It doesn't always go smoothly. It has taken me nearly fifty years to educate my clients to release the head catch first and the squeeze next so that the cow jumps out and turns around to look at me as if to ask, "What the hell was that all about?" When released in the opposite order, a cow backs up and is reluctant to leave. The tests also leave one quite messy with green feces—and I always offer to shake hands with any and all observers. This particular job takes some of the romance out of the profession, but I always tell inquirers that cow manure is green and, to me, it looks and smells like money. They turn up their noses at this statement.

One day I was called to a ranch by a speculator named Don who had purchased one hundred head of heifers. He wanted them pregnancy-tested so he could sell them. I did this job for him and, when finished, gave him the results of the testing: eighty-six head were pregnant.

He looked at me in surprise and said, "That's pretty good for a man who doesn't own a bull."

I assured him that it was very good. In fact, it came close to the average percentile on first-calf heifers. I also told him about another client of mine who had 109 calves out of one neighboring Angus bull that he

PREGNANCY DIAGNOSIS

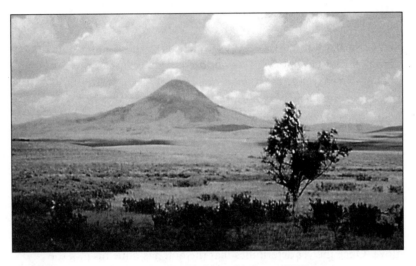

One of the famous Sweetgrass Hills. Photo by Dean Hellinger.

couldn't keep away from his cows. He had all Hereford cows, and when I asked him if he used black bulls on his replacement heifers, he told me that one of his neighbor's Angus yearlings kept jumping the fence. "I would chase him home daily, but his sex drive and libido were such that he would often beat me back before I even finished my daily circle," he had said.

When it finally came time to sell the heifers I had tested, Don put an ad in the paper advertising his great product: "Eighty-six bred heifers, officially preg-tested, ear-tagged, with all shots received. Reasonably priced and ready to go. Please call now."

He received several inquiries and made appointments to show off his herd. All usually went well until the purchaser asked, "What are they bred to?"

Don, being an honest man, would return the question with one of his own. "What do you want them bred to?" he'd ask, showing his willingness to oblige.

The heifers finally found a home, so to speak, and all must have turned out for the good because I never received any bad or good news about the calving results. And Don is still in the cattle brokerage business.

SHORTCUTS

SPRING IS A GLORIOUS TIME in the Golden Triangle. This season when flora and fauna renew themselves is consequently the busiest time of the year for veterinarians. It also has a few drawbacks.

One of these is varied weather. In northern Montana, we get about seventy-five percent of our moisture from March 15 to July 15, before something in the atmosphere disturbs the "El Niño" norm and dries up the whole terrain. Our large state can be treacherously sodden in one area and bone-dry in another. I have always said that Montana is one half-day away from drought and a day away from flood. One of my clients says that when Noah built his ark, it only rained one-eighth of an inch on his place. Other ranchers and farmers brag that it always rains twice as much as anyplace else.

In the first years of my practice here, many of the local roads were neither graveled nor paved. I often faced a dilemma about just which route to take to get to a certain ranch. The long way—which also served as the school bus road—was usually open, but I had one of the no-spin rear-ends, chains, and other things such as snow tires, bigger wheels, and experience to give me an advantage. Nine times out of ten I could usually pull through whatever mud or slush there was on a back route and save time. Being a Swede of the hard-headed variety, I usually took the shortcut.

One fine spring day old Chris Mayer called and left word that two of his two hundred Hereford heifers needed caesarean sections. Each of the cows only weighed about six hundred pounds, had wrinkles—which meant that at one time they had been bigger—and were in bad shape for calving. Chris had run out of hay and his pastures looked like a blade of grass would die of lonesome. To say the least, he was a frugal man. He had an aversion to spending money on either hay or the opposite sex.

Nor did he believe in paying for my services as a veterinarian. I had already delivered about twenty calves for him that spring, mostly by cesarean sections. In order to simplify cost analysis, we had settled on a per-head basis in the past. But I felt that this time, by making two operations on one trip, I might do a little better than just break even.

I pulled into the ranch yard and soon found out that Chris had penned one of the heifers in the ramshackle shed he called a barn. I did the first caesarean in about forty minutes. Then he led me at least five miles out to the pasture where the other heifer was in labor and couldn't move. It was dusk by then, and old Chris was of poor eyesight, so it took us a while to locate the animal.

Meanwhile, I took out my instruments. After we had found the poor creature and secured her in the proper position, I put my tray down and set to work. But Chris meandered around the heifer, taking out his knife to earmark her for future reference, and tripped over my instrument tray. He lost his blade in the process. As he looked for his knife, I redisinfected all of my instruments and began the surgery.

Chris was devastated by his loss and didn't seem to be in complete control. So to keep him from a repeat performance of scattering my instruments, I finally pulled out my good buck knife, handed it to him, and said "Keep the damn thing so I don't have to listen to you bitch anymore." This placated the old boy, and I finally completed the operation.

By then it was dark. We untied all the ropes, which we had tied to our vehicles, and turned the animal loose. She went over and claimed her calf, which was by this time struggling to stand and nurse. We headed back to the ranch house, and in the dark I damn near wiped out the front axle of my car in a couple of badger holes.

My mood wasn't exactly congenial by this time. Besides, some big black rain clouds were moving in from the west, and I was anxious to start for home. I declined Chris's offer of some cowpuncher spuds and headed back toward Conrad—after warning him that he had better spend a little money on hay so that the heifers would milk enough to support their calves until green grass arrived. "A lot of cows and calves die of hollow belly," I told him. I sped along then, leaving a rooster-tail of dust.

Not long after I hit the road, a few raindrops spattered on my windshield. In less than a minute more, I was in the midst of a genuine downpour. I herded my car between the two ditches on either side of the route, hoping the rain would stop before I reached a stretch ominously called Gumbo Flats.

It did. But when I got to Gumbo Flats, I found out why they were so named. Mud built up around my car's wheels until the front wheels would not turn. I couldn't put on chains because the same condition existed with the rear wheels. I was utterly and hopelessly stuck. I couldn't reach anyone on the two-way radio in my rig, so I threw my feather coat down and resigned myself to an evening of slumber.

I woke about daylight. Hoping the soil had dried, I attempted to extricate my trusty vehicle from the mud. In about sixty seconds, I realized that my clutch was no longer functioning. What to do next? I spotted a run-down farm about a mile distant and decided that if its owner had a phone, I could notify someone of my whereabouts. Besides, I was a little hungry by that hour, having missed supper the night before, and was hoping for a little sustenance.

I hadn't walked more than fifty feet when I realized each step was heavier than the one before it. I was packing about thirty pounds of gumbo on each foot—the mud accumulated faster than I could scrape it off. I struggled and cussed. My temperament wasn't improving. I finally reached my destination and found a man named Whirly, an old hermit in a homesteader's shack that hadn't been improved since he had laid claim to it. From Whirly's place I called Chris, and he informed me that he would be down in his Caterpillar tractor to extricate me.

After a hearty breakfast accompanied by an oral accounting of Whirly's lifetime history, Chris's Cat arrived and I was led back to the Mayer place—at the end of a log chain! I performed another caesarean while waiting for help, which finally arrived. I grabbed essential medicines and instruments from my car and got back to Conrad exactly twenty-four hours after I'd left it the day before.

A wrecker towed my car home.

I gave Chris that last caesarean free for towing me—that plus my knife. He tried to talk me out of payment on another call that wet spring, but I wouldn't hear of it. I had figured out that I was already at least three hundred dollars in the hole on his account—and that shortcuts didn't always pay off.

FOUR DAY JOHN

EVERY SO OFTEN a man needs extra help. In spring when calving season is in full swing, and oftentimes in the fall during shipping and roundup times, I worked hard enough to require a few extra hands. When I started out in the morning on those long days, I never knew where I would have to go before I returned home, or what time I would get there. More precise scheduling is one of the benefits—or drawbacks—of better communications. I haven't ever figured out which.

I was running the vet practice out of the ranch and needed a man to watch things when I wasn't around, help feed the cows, plow a few irrigation ditches, watch for calving problems, and even assist me in a caesarean section or two. At last, in desperation, I went down to the state employment office and asked if anyone might be available to help me out.

"Oh, yes," the office staff said. "We have a man waiting out front who would like to go to work right away." The employment officer gave me a two-hour lecture as to salary, hours, working conditions, housing, OSHA, discrimination, affirmative action, and anything else that he deemed pertinent. He then told me that John was just the man I needed. His staff had interviewed him, and they claimed he was as proficient a ranch hand as I liked. He had lived in the country and could take care of things and even cook for himself.

I filled out about ten forms and agreed to meet John that Friday afternoon to take him out and show him around my place. He was waiting for me as appointed. We loaded his gear and headed for the ranch. He was a big, tall man who wore a big straw hat and rolled his own cigarettes. I had been warned never to hire such a man in our windy country because if he wasn't chasing his hat, he was rolling a cigarette. I told him so to break the ice.

He laughed a bit, then said he usually smoked tailor-made Pall Malls, but agreed that he could get along for a few days with Bull Durham.

It was near dinner time when we arrived at our final destination, and I invited him in. Over the meal, he informed me that he wanted Saturday and Sunday to tidy up the house, do his laundry, and get a feel of things. This I agreed to. We parted, and I went to bed.

FOUR DAY JOHN

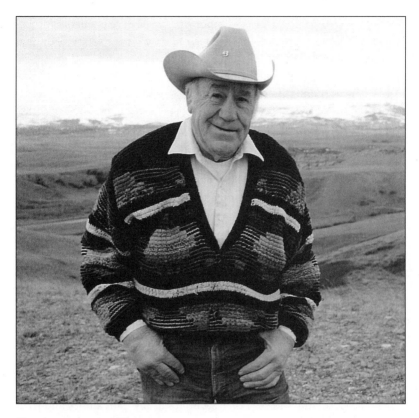

Keeping my sense of humor.

I usually was busy with veterinary work both Saturday and Sunday, since those were the days when all my kids were home from school and available to help with anything else that might be required to be done around the place. If it weren't for weekends and after-school chores, I doubt whether many ranches could survive. Sometimes both ranch parents have outside employment, and I dub them "flashlight farmers" because of the hours they keep. I was no slouch in that department myself—up working for the flashlighters at all hours.

All went well as usual that weekend. The week started off fine. Early Monday morning John presented me with a list of necessities—things he'd need, from toilet paper to light bulbs, groceries, tobacco or cigarettes, gloves, shoelaces, and other sundries I have probably forgotten about. He also needed an advance or draw on his salary for a few other things, such as a "mickey and a six pack," he said.

In order to keep my employee from complaining about abuse, I fulfilled his wishes and said he could ride into town while I went to treat a sick horse with the condition I called "bastard strangles." This is a disease usually starting with a virus syndrome and ending up with a lymphnode streptococcus infection that exhibits itself with great swelling. When the lymph node at last ruptures, copious amounts of evil-smelling yellow pus exude from it. A precursor to respiratory embarrassment, the infection usually requires instant and drastic treatment. Having done my duties, I went to pick up John. I spotted him sniffing the air and the aroma I exuded on the trip home.

It was evening by the time we got home, so we went our separate ways and I didn't see my new employee until the next morning. At seven that morn, he came over to my dwelling and informed me that he didn't think he could fit into the job as well as he thought he might. My tractor didn't have an air-conditioned cab or radio, he said, and he couldn't tolerate the smell and treatment of my client's animals—he had delicate nasal glands. He then asked if I could take him back to town—a duty that the state employment officer had told me was required of an employer.

I said, "Yes," and did so. I then went about my daily duties and tried to catch up with all the lost time. On my rounds, I happened to run into my friend Bill Rumney and told him my sad story.

"You've just been had by 'Four Day John,'" he said. He informed me that John's famous modus operandi was well known all over the territory. He worked the welfare, worker's compensation, and employment systems—plus any potential employers—for all they were worth. I wasn't the only one who had succumbed to the wiles of this charity artist.

Rumney laughed along with me as I echoed P. T. Barnum's famous words, muttering, "There's a sucker born every minute." He then said that I was lucky—he himself had been taken twice. He had also invented the nickname that has since been John's trademark.

COMMON MYTHS DIE HARD

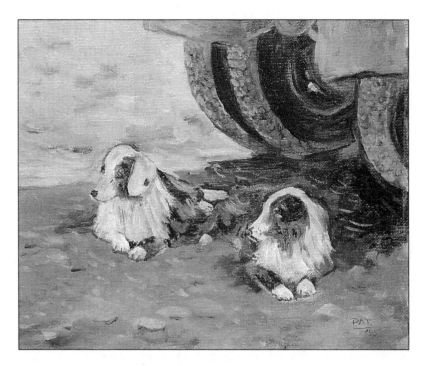

Two cattle dogs with plenty of smarts. Oil painting by Pat Gustafson.

EVER SINCE I CAN REMEMBER, I have listened to people talking about "dumb animals." Well, after years and years of working with animals, I have a profound correction to make: animals are not dumb.

Calling animals dumb could be likened to the former practice of calling deaf people "dumb," just because they wouldn't talk and couldn't communicate in the usual way. We now know better! Hearing loss or a hearing disability has no relation to a low IQ.

On the other hand, I do think some professions show a lack of brainpower—I classify some bankers as having an IQ lower than a snake's ass in a wagon track, and wonder how they ever got through the seventh grade. This is especially true of that goodly number of financial wizards who foreclose on farmers and ranchers who borrowed when prices were high. The bankers can't seem to remember the value of all that collateral they accepted as good enough in the first place. I once threw the keys on

9

one of these bankers' desks and told him, "I did the chores this morning, and if you are going to run the ranch from this desk, it's your turn to do the chores tonight!"

I got off on a tangent there, but now I'll attempt to return to the non-*Homo sapiens* members of the animal kingdom. Animals are not dumb, and they do communicate. My two dogs are smart enough to know the difference between the red and the brown pickup truck. They know when we are moving cattle, and where to be in the process—especially if I tell them. When they have questions about what exactly they're supposed to be doing, they stop and wait for directions. They think ahead, for instance when they sometimes sit on a hill and see if there might be a short cut they can take. They know how to team up to battle a ferocious foe, whether it be badger or raccoon. They know they can't catch a full-grown jack rabbit. They know they're not allowed to chase geese when we're riding along fields or riverbanks. They know they are more than welcome to catch gophers when we are irrigating.

I could go on and on about the intelligence of dogs, but similar things are true for other animals. I don't believe the common notion that most animals are colorblind. Cows aren't, that's for certain. A black bovine will take one look at a red calf and know immediately it isn't hers. Cattle also have clans and pecking orders. They have roles of dominance and timidity. They still know where they have hidden a calf after they have traveled five miles and back to get a drink. They can tell the difference between the hay truck and the "cake" truck. They know exactly where open water is, and when it's time to trail to summer range. They sense when it's time to come home in the fall. "Reluctant" is the word I want to use to describe their attitudes when we head for the corrals at branding time.

Horses have even more smarts. When cutting cattle, they don't want to let one get away anymore than a rider does. They know when you are scared of them. They know when a kid or a greenhorn is riding them. They seem to know when water is too deep to ford. On my ranch, the horses know the dogs and can dodge badger holes better than I can in full canter. They sense when they can get away with something and when they can't.

COMMON MYTHS DIE HARD

Anyone who's spent time with trained horses knows that these special animals often are smarter than their riders. Bulldogging horses know how to run by a steer. Roping horses know how to stop and run backwards, and how to keep a rope tight or ease up when needed. Trail horses learn to pick up a foot so they can be shod. Race horses know how to win a race. I could enumerate so many signs of animal intelligence that writing them down on paper would deplete a whole forest.

Because the so-called dumb beasts are so smart, they sometimes win. One time I observed a cow elk and her calf eluding a hunter. She knew exactly where the hunter was and how to defend herself and the calf against him. It was a game of hide-and-seek, and the hunter never found what he was looking for.

The longer I live, the more I know that I don't know! I have also realized that whatever I've said here about animals, the same can be said about the women in our lives. If you ever think you've got them figured out, you're wrong, wrong, wrong.

THE JET JOCKEY

DURING THE COURSE OF MY PRACTICE I employed students and helpers nearly every year. My helpers were from every veterinary school west of the Mississippi and represented diverse backgrounds. My purpose in hiring them was two-fold: I would learn from them, and they in turn could participate in an active practice and garner a little knowledge of the real world. An additional benefit is that, over the years, some of these helpers have become my friends. And most of the folks who worked with me have gone on to be successful veterinarians in their own right.

Calvin Kelley was one of my one-time assistants. He was the opposite of his namesake, Calvin "Silent Cal" Coolidge, since he could talk the arms and legs off even a complete stranger. Cal especially had the gift of gab or "Irish Blarney" whenever he spotted a beautiful woman.

Although he came from the same generation that I did, Cal's veterinary education had been interrupted by the Korean War. After he made several combat missions and finished his tour of duty as a U.S. Air Force pilot, he was sent back to his home state of Montana to be stationed at Malmstrom Air Force Base in Great Falls. It was from there that he called me, asking if I remembered meeting him in school and on the ski slopes during the years we attended school together. I said that of course I remembered, and invited him to come up and visit anytime he could get away from his military duties. The very next day he showed up and started accompanying me on rural calls and helping around the office.

It was springtime, so I could use all the extra manpower I could get, and Cal proved to be a great assistant. He mixed well with all my clients. He was always in good humor. He even did some baby-sitting on occasion, so my wife and I could get out, and my children loved him.

But Cal had one downfall: booze. He often told me he didn't like to drink just one glass of scotch but would rather down a whole barrelful. I'm certain that this part of his character came out many times at the air base and in the numerous bars in the city of Great Falls.

Oftentimes when he came up to help me he was suffering from the ravages of a hangover. Though he usually wanted to postpone it by having another drink to start out the day, that method didn't coincide with good veterinary practice policy, so instead I would make him suffer. My cure for overindulgence was work. I hoped that, over time, my philoso-

THE JET JOCKEY

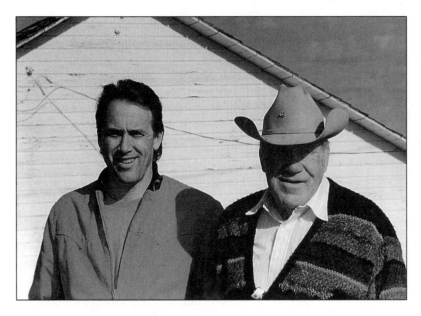

Two musicians: my son Erik "Fingers Ray" and me.

phy on the subject might rub off on him. And for a while it seemed to.

Cal's other indulgences were airplanes and ladies. He seemed right at home among the cattle herds of northern Montana, which were usually made up of females entirely. In order to get more gains and increase the serenity of these cows, ranchers often spayed them, hiring me to remove their ovaries and stop their estrous cycles. This made them focus on finding grass rather than making restless searches for that genuine cowboy, the bull.

That year I had contracted to spay around 3,000 head of females and Cal was to help me. He had taken a week's leave from his duties as a pilot, and we set off to get the job done. We ran through 350 to 400 cattle per day, depending on the circumstances—weather, equipment, etc. The job was quite repetitive and, as a result, boring, so we kept a constant line of chatter—or "bullshit," in the western vernacular—flowing. By the time we finished, we'd passed enough dirty jokes in one ear and out the other to last a lifetime. Only a few of these have stuck with me. One in particular was about a birdwatcher who had found a genuine "Redheaded Double-breasted Mattress Thrasher." I've often wished I could remember more.

After that, whenever the "jet jockey" was on duty, he would fly north and pay us daily visits. He would bless us with everything from sonic booms to flat-hatting maneuvers that would nearly tear the roof off our homes, barns, and outbuildings. It was just Cal's way of saying hello, but I finally had to make him stop such salutations. After a few months, my clients began to call me and complain that their chickens had laid nothing but bloody eggs ever since Cal arrived. The same thing happens when too many chicken hawks get to circling the henhouse.

SEX DRIVE

ALL ANIMALS, *Homo sapiens* included, are the sum of instinct, heredity, and environment. This profound statement can be interpreted in just about any way that scientists, physiologists, or psychiatrists with horse sense want to look at it. I consider it a way of proving that there's little difference between animals and their owners. In all the decades I have practiced veterinary medicine, I rarely have seen a clear line where one begins and the other ends.

I have always loved animals, and have spent my lifetime living with, observing, and training these beautiful creatures. One of my greatest loves is dogs. Every man deserves at least one good one. I have had many good examples of man's best friend: cow dogs, hunting dogs, and even companion dogs that were not particularly good for anything else but companionship. One of my best dogs went by the name of Gus—or, more often, Good Ole Gus. He was darn near human. An Australian shepherd derived from a line of show dogs that had performed all over the world, he also had a bit of border collie in his lineage. I am certain he had an IQ as high as that of some people I know.

Gus was my constant companion for eleven years, often taking the place of several men alongside a cattle chute. He never barked, probably because of the "hush puppy" treatment he'd had during his years of training. In my long days of pregnancy testing or vaccinating six to seven hundred head of cattle, Gus would never quit. As long as I kept water for him beside the chute, he remained at my side waiting to bring the next cow up the line. If there was a creek or water nearby, he would sometimes go for a swim to cool off. But he was always there when I needed him.

Gus was also there for all the neighborhood dogs—he was a prolific breeder. It wasn't long before all the dogs in the area exhibited signs of his lineage. When clients saw him work, they wanted some of his progeny. One day a female was brought in for stud service, and I put them together so they could have a conjugal visit. Gus seemed to enjoy himself immensely.

That night I left Gus in the veterinary hospital room that doubled as a garage and large animal treatment room. This must not have been to his liking, because when I returned at six the next morning he had chewed

15

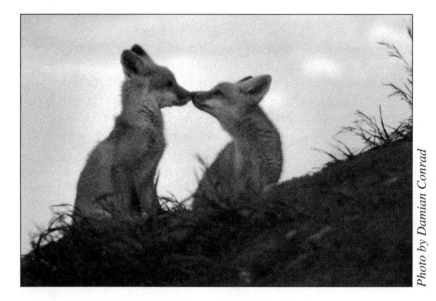

Photo by Damian Conrad

A foxy kiss.

a hole in the tough plastic paneling of the garage door and was sitting patiently outside the steel gate waiting for a second visit with his newfound friend.

That's what I call sex drive.

It isn't much different when a stallion is about to be taken out of his stall to service a mare. Horses have extra-sensory perception when this occurs, and the stallions nearly go frantic. Their neighing and flatulence has been mimicked by comedians in the agricultural field for as many years as I can recall. I miss the days of the explosive fart and ecstatic squeal of a stallion in the anticipation of a little sex.

Cattle are no different. Bulls can cut out a harem of cows and separate them as quickly as a stallion guarding his band on the open range. And wild animals are the same. A good imitated elk bugle can make a bull respond by crashing through timber, looking for an intruder. Rattling deer horns can bring in a competing buck or a few hopeful does. The dance of pintail grouse brings in hens, as does the crow of a rooster. A gander and his goose keep in close touch with their mating calls.

SEX DRIVE

But sex drive isn't limited to animals. The women of our own species decorate themselves with lipstick, jewelry, perfume, and other accoutrements to attract men. I particularly like the short skirts. It's a competitive field—I think I had to take my wife home once just because she spotted someone who was wearing a dress just like the one she had on. I could also talk about the men who tipple a few and think they are God's gift to women. I can recall one time in high school that I had a few beers and got a little fresh with a pretty Norwegian girl. She reached over and hit me, giving me a nosebleed. This interrupted all thoughts of romance.

Shakespeare made a classic statement about just such a case when writing about the relationship of alcohol to sex. "It increases the desire," he said, "but inhibits the performance." I guess I had better shut up on the subject, since this is supposed to be a book about animals. I will never understand all the aspects of sex drive, but I know that from the beginning of time it has occupied the time and energy of all creatures, human and otherwise.

RESTRAINT

RESTRAINT IS NINETY PERCENT of veterinary medicine. In order to get any job done properly, whether it be an operation on a buffalo or a canary, the patient must be held in such a way that it can be treated with whatever procedure is required to return it to a healthy status. Needless to say, this isn't always easy.

Buffalo are restrained in a way that's similar to how we treat cattle. They can be caught in a squeeze chute, although one has to be more wary of their ominous horns and head. Once they are securely caught, we test them for most of the diseases common to bovines. We inseminate, pregnancy-test, castrate, dehorn, and even in some instances brand them. By the time most of these procedures are completed, a bison's temperament has changed to that of an irate female. I wouldn't recommend standing in front of the chute when one is released.

Buffalo are no worse than Brahma bulls, though. A Brahma is by far the most agile and difficult animal to ride, which is why it takes such a place in most rodeos. When matched against even the best of cowboys, the bull generally wins. Bull-riding is still one of the most dangerous sports event there is—ski jumping is tame in comparison.

Some cats refuse to be restrained, and most cats are difficult to hold and treat. Every vet or cat owner has probably been on the receiving end of feline endeavors to extricate themselves. Scratches and bites are usually the way it goes. Most of the time the cat wins. It is much easier to anesthetize a cat than nurse deep wounds.

For some reason cats and dogs often are not compatible, and the inherent fear of a cat for a dog has caused pandemonium and catastrophic results in many a crowded waiting room. When a cat's eyes get about the size of old silver dollars, it's time to move the poor thing into another waiting room so it doesn't scratch the neck, arms, or mammary glands of the owner or a brave assistant.

Speaking of felines, I can recall one day that one of my clients from the "cat house" in a neighboring town brought in a toy breed that resembled a rag mop to be spayed. Several days later, as arranged, a couple of the girls came in to pick up their darling. I don't know what happened, but the smell of their perfume must have stimulated little Rag Mop's instincts. As my faithful assistant was retrieving her from the cage, the dog squirmed out of her arms and hit the floor running.

About the same time, Emory, who was a large, lumbering farmer, walked in the door—opening Rag Mop's escape route. My secretary Barbara, who was dressed in a white uniform and open-toed sandals, took after the precious beast, but by that time the smell of pigs and manure emanating from Emory's presence must have added olfactory fuel to Rag Mop's engines. In spite of her mistresses' distressing calls, she did not stop.

Not until she hit the road in front of my office, that is. There, the highway department was spreading fresh tar. The immaculate white dog headed directly for the gooey black mess, with my white-clad assistant in swift pursuit. The envisioned result occurred. Rag Mop ran through an extra thick puddle of petroleum-based pavement before Barbara could capture her and clasp her tightly to her bosom.

When faithful assistant and escapee returned to the office, both appeared quite different. Barbara's sandals and uniform made her look like one of my clients' black-and-white pinto horses. Rag Mop was no longer immaculately groomed and clean, but resembled a tarred-and-feathered felon from the olden days.

I sent Barbara home with alcohol and acetone and it was decided that the little dog, if you could call it that, should be cleansed before returning to the local "wild-life sanctuary," as we called it. It took about four days of intensive cleansing with various solvents, cleansing agents, and detergents, and numerous baths, combings, and brushings before Rag Mop returned to her original appearance. But, as I said before, animals are not dumb—she'd learned from her mistake. When it was finally time to return home to Roxie's House on the Hill, Rag Mop made no second attempt to escape from the confines of the clinic.

And I am reasonably certain that she spent the rest of her life in a perfumed atmosphere.

I FORGOT MORE THAN YOU'LL EVER
KNOW ABOUT HORSES

HORSES HAVE BEEN IMPORTANT TO ME ever since I was old enough to straddle one. My affection for the animals has led me to look into their history in the Golden Triangle region, and I have discovered that the equine species arrived in Montana for the first time around 1734. The arrival of this stately animal greatly changed the history of our area, which until that time had remained more or less static since its first humans arrived.

The Blackfeet people, who lived here before the horses came, had quite limited modes of transportation. They packed all their belongings on their back or loaded them on travois pulled by domesticated wolf-dogs. They hunted bison on foot, enticing the giant beasts over cliffs called *pishkuns* or buffalo jumps. After brave decoys dressed in wolf skins drove the buffalo in the general direction of a pishkun, other tribal members waved blankets and hides to scare the herd over the precipice to their demise.

This method of getting food and buffalo hides was changed by the arrival of the horse, which the Blackfeet named an "elk-dog." Mounted on horses, "buffalo runners" could travel alongside a stampeding bison herd, firing arrows into the animals' rib cages. The entire tribe was enlisted in butchering the resulting lines of dead or injured buffalo, and the carcasses were transported back to Indian encampments by horsepower. The Blackfeet soon developed a Plains Indian culture, with increased mobility.

A little more than one hundred years later, the same sea of grass that fed the buffalo and Blackfeet horses tempted new speculators and cowboys. As these men trailed cattle north to Montana from Texas and California, the horse again garnered the spotlight. Because the horse was the animal of choice to control vast cattle herds, its use developed by leaps and bounds. Horses helped when cattle were branded, trailed, shipped, rounded-up, and marked for various owners. Horse remudas of as many as five hundred head accompanied the round-ups. These great traveling horses often were derived from Justin Morgan's draft horses crossed with native mustangs, along with Thoroughbreds brought in for great speed or colorful Nez Perce and Shoshone appaloosas. Their ability, stamina, and skill made the cowboy and his horse inseparable.

The old-fashioned livery stable was one of the focal points of the horse business. There, horses were rented, traded, bought, sold, shod, fed, housed, and treated for disease. Tack was repaired, harnesses made, and wagon wheels rimmed with metal. A livery stable was one of the busiest places in all frontier settlements—outside myth, it was probably frequented more than the romantic saloon. Here people gathered to hash and rehash stories of horses and training methods, and events such as a ride across a wintry prairie were exaggerated like the fish tales of our day.

Later, homesteaders flocked to Montana with the team, wagon, and plow. They broke up the sod, lived, and perished under searing sun, dust storms, droughts, and insect plagues. In those early days, farm work was done by equine power. The logging industry used draft teams to deliver their product to the sawmills. Old photographs show draft teams with as many as thirty horses used to build the railroads, roads, and dams that later made real horsepower obsolete.

The prolific, horsey West soon began producing specialty horses for the affluent East: polo ponies, hunters, jumpers, and even an occasional racehorse (such as the famous Kentucky Derby winner Spokane, raised by Montana's copper king Marcus Daly). Montana and the West also produced many of the horses used by the U.S. Cavalry.

When times turned bad in the droughty 1920s, the exodus of thousands of homesteaders left the Montana range full of unwanted horses. These were the beginnings of many of the wild horse herds we sometimes still see here today. Many were rounded up and used as animal and fish feeds, dog food, and today for human consumption in Europe and Third World countries. Going back sixty years or so, I can recall the Cremer Rodeo Company trailing horse herds from the Crazy Mountains to Billings, Montana, where Leo Cremer was the livestock contractor for the Midland Empire Fair.

In 1935, my brothers and I trailed the remnants of our horse herd from Rapelje to Bozeman. Our grubstake at that time was a "roll of red and a loaf of bread." My brother raided a chicken house one morning, so we had a fried-egg breakfast and a few hard-boiled eggs left over for a welcome dietary change.

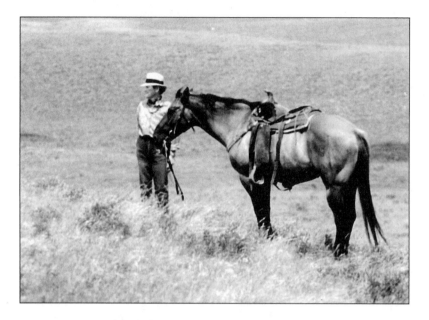

Friend Pat and her horse on a trail drive.

One day when I was very young, while rounding up some of the semi-wild horses near our homestead, I pulled up my horse short and lost the herd. Just then, my dad pulled up, too—in his Model-A Ford. He pulled out a lariat and massaged my butt a couple of times. Then he asked, "Do you think you can turn those horses now?"

"Yes," I said. Now, every time I think I might lose a herd of either horses or cattle, I recall the lesson and try harder. Over the years it has paid off.

One of the first ranches that I worked on, at twelve years of age, trailed its horses from Ennis, Montana, to Reynolds Pass on the Idaho border. We would leave at daylight and take off at the most natural gait of a horse, a trot. During lunch break, after fording the Madison River, we changed horses. We arrived at our destination, sixty to seventy miles distant, at about four in the afternoon. I remember another annual trail drive from near Boulder, Montana, to the Upper Madison thirty miles south of Ennis before the advent of World War II. Some people think of some of these trail drives as romantic, and call me lucky. Maybe so, but I can still recall how boring it was to a youngster to look at the "ass end" of a cow, day after day. With all the trailing I've done in my life, I didn't feel much like participating in the great Centennial Cattle Drive from Roundup to Billings in 1989.

Modern and improved transportation has changed the livestock industry so much that our ancestors would hardly recognize it. Today, instead of animals transporting the human population, we transport them in trains, trucks, and livestock trailers, just as if they are family members.

I've spent a good deal of time in the saddle. I broke and trained all the rope horses, dogging horses, and ranch horses we used on our ranch. I feel qualified as a has-been rancher, veterinarian, and rodeo participant to pass on my thoughts about the breaking and training process.

There are thousands of methods and means of training a horse. Many of these have been handed down for centuries by the trainers of war horses, chariot horses, stagecoach horses, draft horses, pack horses, racehorses, and livery horses broken for diversified reasons. Any good trainer learns early that a person has to be smarter than the animal he or she wants to teach, helping the horse develop good habits rather than bad ones. For instance, in halter breaking, a horse learns to step forward to relieve the pressure of the halter on his head. If a horse caused the rope to break when he resisted, or if it came untied before the halter was properly introduced, it would learn instead to pull back—and doing so would become a chronic bad habit.

I usually started breaking all my horses as two-year-olds. They ran free in pastures from the time they were weaned, branded, and halter-broke. In the spring of their second year, they were brought in to be castrated or spayed, according to my desires of the times. After a healing period of two weeks, I would halter them, tie them, and hobble the one or two that I would begin to train.

After saddling both horses, I would take them on a mile-long ride, using a pony lead. I would then put on a hackamore and tie each horse's head around to the rear D-ring on the back cinch. Their conditioned reflexes soon ruled. After circling a few times, they learned to give their head to the pressure of the hackamore.

Then came the time for the first mounting. I believe a trainer can do more in ten minutes on top of a horse than he or she can accomplish in two or three days of ground work. In a very small round or square corral, I pulled the horse's head around, intertwining my hand in the mane so that I could tighten the inside rein if necessary. Then, in one fluid motion, I got on, staying as close to the horse as possible. This procedure was usually eventless, especially in a small corral where the horse could not run or get away.

Once on top, I began to teach the horse to move forward under a loose rein and to stop when pressure is applied to the nose with a hackamore (or mouth pressure, if a snaffle bit is used). This again applied conditioned reflexes, and repetition was of the essence. Using a hair rein or mecate with the slightest of pressure caused enough skin sensation that a horse was usually neck reining in four or five training sessions.

Other examples of good horse sense? Always make a horse under halter come up to you instead of you walking up to him—otherwise he may back up all over the barnyard while you try to get up to him. The so-called whip breaking of a horse is nothing more than conditioning him to react to the sting of a whip every time he turns his head away from you. An animal soon learns that pain or annoyance stops when he keeps his head turned in the right direction. But the rewards of petting and kindness are much better than the alternatives; the old saying that honey will catch more flies than vinegar holds true. Finally, repetition is the essence of training. Reining horses, roping horses, barrel-racing horses, and cutting horses are made to repeat proper procedures thousands of times before they become the champion performers we see in the arena. Rodeo has brought about the introduction of more good horses than any other factor.

After serving as a judge of horseflesh for nearly half a century I have seen all colors, shapes, sizes, and breeds. To each his own—but I am prejudiced to quarter horses. My family imported some of the first quarter horses into Montana in 1939. They came from Texas, where they were developed by the settlers who took their best horses to that country after the chaos of the Civil War. It was here that Steel Dust, Zantanon,

Peter McCue, and other early sires of the breed left their mark. Many were scattered throughout the west when the great trail herds moved north. Quarter horses are famous for their versatility and great speed at short distances. The proof is in the pudding—the quarter horse list is the largest breed registry in the world. There are many types within the breed by adapting the best of the Thoroughbred, Arab, Morgan, and even heavier draft breeds.

I've never known a man who thought that the horse he owned was not the best.

This is especially true when it comes to horse racing. I can't recall all the alibis and rationalizations that have been passed on to me as to why a favorite steed didn't win a race or do incredibly well in other endeavors of competition. Racehorse men usually live with their horses and develop spectacular attachments to them. They have to be fed at daylight, kept in impeccably clean stalls, and exercised and trained daily. Winning just one race seems to solidify this lifelong bond. Oftentimes, a beloved animal is retained well past his prime competitive years. I have seldom known a racehorse owner who didn't think a certain feed additive, medicine, or drug wouldn't give his favorite the stamina of youth, so he could keep on winning a few more times before he would be put out to pasture.

For many years, I was the veterinarian at our racetrack in Shelby, Montana. It is one of many so-called "bush" tracks that are borderline in both number of races and prize money awarded. A regular circuit established in the surrounding towns and counties enables an owner or trainer to keep a stable of ponies for the entire racing season. As veterinarian, I was responsible to see that all race prospects were physically fit and free of drugs so as not to endanger the life of the animal or the jockey—and so that all concerned had an equal chance.

We routinely collected urine or blood samples. However, no matter how many rules were promulgated, there always seemed to be a loophole that would cover up some performance drugs or illegal feeds. A few trainers and owners had different tricks of the trade up their sleeve— they were always willing to try for a win, even though cheating might mean a hearing before the state gaming commission or a possible suspension of their privileges.

My old friend Avery, who had been around horses and racetracks since he was knee-high to a grasshopper, was just such a person. He was a great "Doctor Bell's" man. "Doctor Bell's" is a potent liquid that contains the drug atropine. An effective euphoric drug, a favorite of many racehorse owners, it could only be purchased in Canada without prescription. The usual dosage was one or two drops on the tongue of a horse, used for any number of equine ailments, including certain types of colics. In some ailments, it serves as a placebo—more for the owner than for the horse.

Avery had an elderly horse who had been nominated for non-winners, and I'm certain he gave that favorite of his more than a fair share of "Doctor Bell's." Although another veterinarian had been employed by the gaming commission at that time, I just happened to be around when Avery's race was called. I didn't get to lean over the rail to watch, but it wasn't long before Avery was leading his horse, named By-a-Nose, back to the stables. I called out to him, inquiring how he had finished. His instant reply was, "He didn't win, but he was the happiest son-of-a-bitch loser out there!"

I brought up five of my own kids on horseback, without many undue hazards or accidents—that is, not too many until I got the desire to add too much racehorse breeding to my bloodlines. Like Avery, I ended up with horses that were ultimately unsatisfactory for my desires and needs. I'm now on my way back to the day when I had just the stock I needed and was ignorant enough to not know it. Today, I want a horse that is born broke, has lots of cow sense, is pretty to look at, easy to ride, and gentle, and has the confirmation to carry me all day on a round-up or cattle drive.

Most of all, I want one I can trust to put my grandchildren on without fearing that their lives are in jeopardy. I'd like a horse that can carry a seven- or eight-year-old grandson as we head out to a lake full of fish or start up the trail to summer pasture. I'd be happy with a horse that we both could climb on and ride around, just for the fun of it.

HERSHEL

HERSHEL WAS A SAINT BERNARD of even greater proportions than the average. I had been associated with him ever since he was six weeks old, when he was presented to me as an awkward puppy for his usual inoculations. From puppyhood, he was an exuberant animal, and often knocked over loose objects with his massive tail or huge paws. He slobbered constantly from his flopping jowls.

After Hershel's first visit to my office, his owner Steve placed him in the cab of his pickup and the two drove off. It was not long afterward that he returned for his second series of inoculations and rabies vaccination. By that time, Hershel wasn't riding in the cab—he was standing in the truck bed, tall as the cab itself, taking in the gorgeous views. Steve said that his charge attracted roadside dogs during his daily travels, moving first from one side of the pickup box to the other. It had made driving more difficult.

It wasn't long before Hershel's first catastrophe—he cut his paw on a piece of glass and was delivered to the animal hospital covered with gore. One toe was nearly severed, with half of the footpad nearly cut off. Blood was still spurting from the wound as I unloaded him into the large-animal portion of our hospital, knowing he would not fit on the small-animal examination table. I gave him general anesthesia and, quickly as I could, repaired his wounds. Putting on several layers of bandages, I covered his entire foot and half the leg, then moved him to a large pen for a day or two of recovery. Soon he was riding around in Steve's pickup as before, viewing the grand scenery of the Rocky Mountain Front and its beautiful snowcapped peaks.

Hershel's next visit to the hospital was for a broken and ulcerated tail. Since neither the fracture or the ulcer was healing correctly, my partner removed half of the Saint Bernard's tail. But Hershel would not leave what was left of his massive appendage alone. He kept biting and licking it until nearly all that was left of the tail was a huge, ulcerative wound.

To correct the condition, I had no choice but to remove the entire tail. After the operation, I put a big inner tube around bobtailed Hershel's neck in order to prevent a repeat of his own canine treatment. Again, healing was uneventful, and Hershel got back to the business of riding in

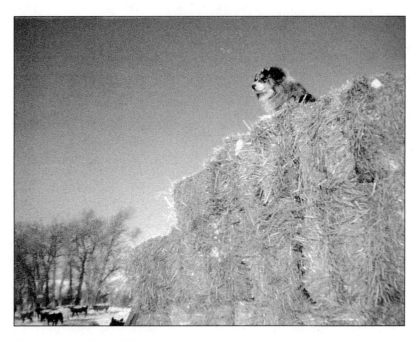

The overseer of the bale wagon.

the rear end of a truck, surveying hill and dale. He looked a bit odd without a large tail wagging behind him.

The operation had an unforeseen result—the drastic removal of the dog's important appendage also changed his temperament. Since Hershel had not even a stub to wag at other dogs, he found other endeavors meant to impress them. These didn't afford him any human benevolence, though. In his wanderings one day he came upon a neighbor's farrowing yard full of young piglets and developed a taste for fresh pork. Steve paid for a litter of pigs not once but twice.

But the third time Hershel ate pig, Steve's neighbor decided the Saint Bernard was no saint. He was incorrigible, it seemed, and met an untimely demise, dying of lead poisoning from the irate neighbor's gun.

FADS

FADS ARE AS COMMON in the animal world as fashions in New York or new hairstyles in high school. Everyone wants to be different, never giving a thought to practicality. Through the processes of genetic engineering, we have spotted asses, miniature pigs that won't even make good chop suey, miniature horses that do little more than defecate, Shitzu dogs that are so wrinkled that even a veterinarian has trouble deciding which end to work on, and Lhasa Apso lap dogs that look like automated mops. These are just a few anomalies of the animal world. The old saying that diversity is the spice of life keeps a veterinarian on his toes, since specific syndromes are prevalent in each animal species and breed. This is probably one of the reasons that admission to veterinary school is so difficult.

My observation is that most of these fads are started by someone with a monetary goal. Once the novelty of an exotic animal wears thin, or the novelty's owner grows tired of following the creature around with a "pooper-scooper," the pets end up in a veterinary hospital. I have been chastised many times for my numerous suggestions that we develop sprays similar to pesticides or herbicides for those pets that have become unloved and unwanted, having lost their value as a topic of conversation.

But other pets are wanted until the end. I recall the day that an elderly lady presented me with a pet of hers, suffering from a terminal illness. It obliged me by terminating on the examination table while I was checking its vital signs. I went out to inform the client of her pet's demise and had no more than looked at her when she broke into convulsive sobbing. I did my best to console her, but was of little avail. She cried for about thirty minutes.

When we finally arrived at a communicative level, I informed her that her lifelong friend had died from cumulative congestion of the arteries, from circulatory failure—and senility. She seemed to be satisfied with this explanation, although she made one last statement that I'll never forget. As she gathered her composure and turned to leave, she said, "I think I would have just as soon lost my husband as poor little Fifi."

VENTILATION

WE ARE PRETTY WELL VENTILATED here in Northern Montana, where wind usually blows in a counter-clockwise movement. The upslope movement along the Rocky Mountain Front causes the atmosphere to cool down, and moisture is the result. We don't receive a lot of moisture on a yearly basis at our ranch, usually from thirteen to fifteen inches a year, but thirty-five miles west, on the Continental Divide, they get thirty to thirty-five inches of rain or snowfall.

Timing of this water drop is of the utmost importance. We receive most of our moisture from April to mid-July, which is our growing season, with long days and short nights. The moisture makes grass for animals and adds essential water to the irrigation reservoirs on one of the greatest bread baskets of the nation. Because of its sensitive nature, weather is always foremost in the minds of nearly everyone in the livestock and related agribusinesses here.

Wind is the one weather feature that's constant. Ninety percent of the time the southwest to northeast runways at local airports are the only ones used. If wind power is ever harnessed to its potential, our local development of this natural resource will be boundless. Until then, we'll have to let it use up its own strength—blowing railroad cars off the tracks and tipping over high-profile vehicles.

My own encounters with the wind have been many. One day while traveling down the highway, I thought I had encountered some alien objects. But it was only a convoy of motorcyclists leaning into the wind at a 45-degree angle. After a few gusts, they turned tail and returned to the nearest town to await more favorable conditions. I hoped they would spread rumors about the bad Montana weather.

In one of our good winds, guns won't shoot straight. Don't expectorate or micturate into the breeze. Forgo straw hats, smoking, or attempting to walk into the gusts. If it's snowing and blowing, make certain you're driving on an elevated road, because a good ground blizzard can drift into cuts and gullies and close a wide highway in minutes.

I can't think of many incidents where I relished the wind, which seems to be more severe in fall and early spring. March, a cattle man's busiest time of year, usually brings on some of the greatest velocities. The breeze can blow the real estate here back and forth so many times in a dry year that no one can really claim to own land.

One day I was returning from a call near the town of Dupuyer. I had been going night and day for about two days and had neglected to read the gauges in front of my eyes that inform one of the amount of fuel left to run the engine. Via two-way radio, the folks in my office said that many important emergency calls were awaiting my return. By dead reckoning I told them I should be there in about ten minutes. Time is of the essence in veterinary medicine, especially in O.B. cases, prolapses, milk fevers, bloats, etcetera.

I was just returning from replacing a uterine prolapse on a wild-eyed 1,600 pound Charolais cow, which had been uncooperative. The process had left neither me nor she in a good temperament—I had the disposition of a German shepherd with a mouthful of porcupine quills. About 6 miles west of town, just before the downgrade of Sam George Hill, my engine sputtered and quit.

Since I had only one little rise to surmount, I hoped that I could coast over it and make it into town. A strong wind was blowing behind me at about 70 miles per hour, but my speed gradually decreased and I didn't think I could make it over the last little hump. Then I opened the door of my sedan, thinking I could jump out and help with a little push. But the door on a two-door sedan in those days was about five feet long, and it made a decent windsail. The minute I opened the door, the car began to pick up speed. I immediately reached over and popped open the other door, realizing then and there that other men's dreams of propelling ships, covered wagons, and even Lewis and Clark in their portage around the Great Falls of the Missouri by wind had some validity. I coasted right up to the gas station under natural power, and my temperament improved. I made it through the day thinking about my turn in fortune, and ever since that day have been a little more tolerant of the air currents.

The only time I lost faith in the atmosphere was when an 80-mile-an-hour gust ripped my ear-flapped Scotch cap off my head and sent it skidding over thin ice until it caught in a bunch of cattails, along with beer and pop cans. I couldn't get to it, and spent the rest of the day bareheaded in misery, accumulating a new vocabulary with which I could vent my frustration about over-ventilation.

ROCKY MOUNTAIN OYSTERS

THE ROCKY MOUNTAIN OYSTER is indeed an endangered species. There is not a "branding bee" that goes by in our area that he is not attacked and his species diminished to the last morsel. Half of the requests I get from friends and acquaintances are to "save the gonads for me."

Perhaps I should explain what a Rocky Mountain oyster is. During branding, young bull calves are neutered and the disembodied testicles are what we refer to as sea creatures. These real ranch land treats are cooked up and served as hors d'oeuvres at high-society cocktail parties and skid row bars. At local rodeos and cowboy golf tournaments or anywhere else festive, they can be obtained in sufficient quantities to please.

The "oysters" are prepared in a variety of ways. Some are consumed fresh and pronto, after being laid atop the branding stove and turned until they pop like popcorn. Others are cleaned and deep frozen, dipped in pancake batter or rolled in corn and cereal meals laced with spices and pepper. They go good with beer or any other type of cocktails.

Known as an aphrodisiac of sorts, they are served to "pilgrims" and squeamish diners without their knowledge and are indeed conversational ice breakers. New girlfriends or boyfriends who have never tasted them are usually forced to defend themselves by taking the first nibble after seeing plate after plate disappear under the grasping talons of gluttonous aficionados.

I don't think the misnamed oysters have been indicted yet for coliform or ptomaine toxicity, but only since cowboys carry a natural immunity to such organisms or else quell their proliferation with alcohol and beer. One of my friends was prohibited from serving what are also called "calf fries" next to the beer concession at our local rodeo one time, since they had not been inspected and passed on by the federal government. The inspector confiscated them, but pleaded the Fifth Amendment when I asked him to verify their disposal.

I doubt that the testosterone content of a Rocky Mountain oyster has ever been evaluated. I am not so wise as these lawyer guys, but it's my opinion that the beer and whiskey make more monkeys out of cowboys than do the famous oysters. A meal of these fries might get a ranch hand's sex drive in gear or his hormones clanking, but I can't tell where

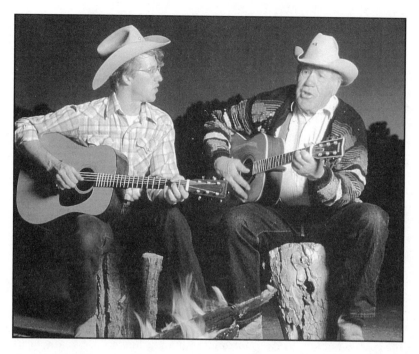

Once in a while Wylie still lets me sing.

instinct stops and environment takes over. Better advice against this kind of vice has been offered by the famous western singer who said, "Mamma, don't let your boys grow up to be cowboys."

MOUSE AND PICKLES

I CAN'T GUARANTEE THE AUTHENTICITY of this story about two of my neighbors, but I can't find any reason to disbelieve it either.

Mouse and Pickles were bronc riders of renown in their early days, two brothers who were remembered in part because of their nicknames— not many people have similar handles. The men owned a string of bucking horses and contracted with local rodeo producers to furnish some or most of the rough stock.

One year, the two boys took a contract to supply the bucking horses for a rodeo in Fort Benton. The producer told them he would furnish the transportation to get them there. I don't know the other details of their contract, but their pay must have been based on a percentage of the gate transaction. It seemed like a fair deal to Mouse and Pickles, but the boys didn't reckon according to Murphy's famous law, which says that whatever can possibly go wrong, will.

It did. One of Montana's many rain and hail storms materialized and wiped out any chance of rodeo attendance—and thus, the receipts. Since the contractor didn't have any money, and since there was no clause in the contract about his transporting the animals home, Mouse and Pickles were on their own. They decided to go the cheap route and trail them home.

Plans were made to start early the next morning. The two men purchased a couple of loaves of bread, a couple of rolls of bologna, and a couple of gallons of Thunderbird wine—plus a magnum of rotgut whiskey apiece. Before they left for the trail, the brothers made an agreement that they wouldn't drink any of this latter supply, but planned to sell or bootleg it on the nearby reservation to help restore their financial status.

After their early start the brothers were unusually sober, due to their empty wallets and the fact that they had more than a hundred miles to go before returning to their ranch headquarters on Badger Creek. The trail was dusty, and the weather was hot. They met one man on the way, a son of the soil who stopped them and chewed the fat for a spell. They drained his water jug as he told them that the big rain and hail storm had just missed that part of the country, so they'd probably have a dry trail until they hit the dry fork of the Marias River. After this bit of information, the farmer told the boys he was damn dry himself—and

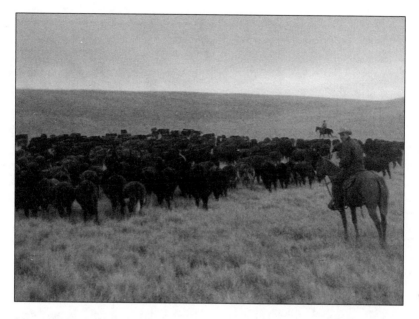

Moving a herd to market.

would give anything for a "good" drink.

Mouse's brain cells really started working then. He offered the gentleman a shot of whiskey and a chaser of wine for a dollar. His offer was readily accepted, the liquor poured, and Mouse tucked the silver dollar into his pants pocket. They continued on their way.

True to its name, and as the farmer had said, the Dry Fork was dry—as a bone. The prospect of staking a dry camp with only a roll of red and a loaf of bread was catastrophic—the brothers looked around but couldn't find a drop of anything to wash a mouthful of supper down. Then another thought hit Mouse like a bolt of lightning. "Pickles," he said, "I have a dollar. Would you sell me a shot of whiskey and a chaser of wine?"

"Certainly," said Pickles. "It wouldn't be breaking our agreement of not giving any booze away or drinking any of our own personal supply." And so the sale was completed.

Now Pickles had the silver dollar. Money seems to burn a hole in certain people's pockets, and Pickles was never known to be a miser.

"Mouse," he began, "you wouldn't mind selling me a double shot with a chaser for a dollar, would you?"

The two dined fabulously on bread and bologna, complimenting the fare as the silver dollar went back and forth as each sale was made. A final after-dinner drink ended their great feast, and they fell into a euphoric slumber until the rays of a rising sun and a howling pack of coyotes aroused them and started them on their way.

Their next planned stop was a place called Sober Up Creek, right near "Molly's Nipple," a prominent butte only a few miles from home. During the course of the day, they sold quite a lot of whiskey, exchanging the silver dollar back and forth. By the time they hit water on Sober Up Creek, their horses were sore-footed and thirsty. They took on a fill of water and began to load up on good lupine and grass.

Pickles and Mouse also took a fill and a rest. They finished off the bread and the red, sold the rest of the booze, and tanked up on Sober Up water. Since there was no one around, they slept real good. They arrived home early the next day.

They're successful ranchers now. To this day, neither one has mentioned a thing to the other about the whiskey profits.

LOCKJAW

LOCKJAW IS THE COMMON TERM for tetanus. It is a disease that affects many animals, including humans, and once the symptoms appear, death usually follows. It is a first cousin to blackleg, malignant edema, septicemia, and many other diseases caused by the clostridial group.

Most of us have experienced some of the pains people take to prevent lockjaw. Every time you or one of your children stepped on a nail or had an accident that caused a deep puncture wound, you were rushed to the doctor and soon found yourself on the burning end of a painful rear-end shot—after unceremoniously dropping your britches so the doctor or nurse could get a good run at that good round target. Besides being nauseated from the thought of just getting a tetanus booster shot, you would be extremely sore for a few days from its effects. The reason for the embarrassing precaution is that the disease is no joking matter.

In all my years as a veterinarian, I have been on the lookout for this condition. The most common occurrence is in lambs after they have been castrated and had their tails docked. It also appears occasionally in calves and young foals, contracted from umbilical infection at birth or shortly thereafter. The disease is sometimes seen in older animals after castration or surgery, and we treat it today by routinely giving tetanus antitoxin after most operations to avoid litigation.

But there is a more humorous aspect of the term lockjaw, which doesn't necessarily refer to the disease. What I call lockjaw also occurs when a horse gets a rope under his tail. The tail on a horse is a muscular contraption that can be as tightly squeezed as a vise. When this happens, and the horse turns to see what is stuck on his anal sphincter, a secondary symptom of severe rope burn is inflicted. This causes even more emotional stress on the poor animal and an immediate and instant reflex that isn't as benign as the knee jerk reflex an M.D. uses to test human reflexes on an insurance examination.

The horse begins to fight. I mean *really* fight. I have seen entire packstrings get away and spread their drover's gear over a mountainside. I have seen branding crews wiped out. I have seen many cowboys pick themselves out of the corral dust asking, "What the hell happened?" All kinds of pandemonium can result from this lockjaw syndrome. The safest place is high on the corral fence or completely over it.

LOCKJAW

After going completely mad, some horses lose any degree of sanity and remain that way for the remainder of their lives. Others can be cured by the Crupper Method, which requires that the horse become used to a strange apparatus close to its prurient parts.

Anybody that has been around horses or animals an entire life knows that it's not the best solution. Avoid lockjaw at all costs.

SHIT COULEE

JIM CALLED ME FROM a bar about midnight and asked me when I could castrate his mules. I wasn't too tickled about setting up an appointment at that time of the night and asked why it was imperative that we make our appointment at such a time. "Well," he said, "I just got to thinking that if I cut those mules myself they will hate me for the rest of their lives." I told him to go home, go to bed, sober up, and bring the mules down first thing in the morning.

I didn't know if he would remember, so I called him at six the next morning to remind him of the appointment. He arrived at about 8:30, and I invited him in for a cup of coffee. Before we went out to do the work, we reminisced about times gone by. Jim was just a little whippersnapper when I first knew him. His dad was a local banker and livestock trader from time to time. He had purchased a little piece of ground to feed his livestock, trading bulls, saddle horses, a few pigs, and other animals he bought until they could be sold or traded.

Earl, Jim's dad, had put up some ramshackle corrals and a few buildings along a little stream just north of town that ran out of the Turd Lakes—our name for the sewer lagoons constructed by the town. For that reason, we called the place Shit Coulee.

When Jim finally finished high school, his dad had big plans for his future. He gave Jim $2,500 and sent him to Bozeman, site of Montana State University, to further his education. But Jim and higher education were like oil and water—they didn't mix. Jim spent a glorious ninety days spending the fortune, but I doubt if he ever exposed himself to a classroom. Anyway, that ended his—or his father's—aspirations for higher education. Jim returned home to Conrad, moved a small shack out to Shit Coulee to continue his lifestyle of beer and whiskey consumption.

In my travels, I would often find Jim passed out along the road on a Sunday morning or looking for a ride to some destination where he could find a beer to postpone a hangover. He finally migrated to the Blackfeet Indian Reservation, where he met and married a beautiful woman by the name of Lorretta Bull Shoe, who was from a well-known family living close to Heart Butte. They set up a small ranch raising horses, cattle, and hay, and he still resides there to this day. I've done veterinary work for them from time to time.

SHIT COULEE

I castrated Jim's mules in spite of his fears. Today he uses them in his yearly hunting trips to the Bob Marshall Wilderness, where he sets up his tepee and spends a month or two in the "Big Rock Candy Mountains," where there is plenty of room to roam.

Last year, however he told me that after one of his escapades and his ninth ticket for Driving Under the Influence, they had put a radio collar on him and sent him back to the ranch under house arrest. He petitioned to have the collar removed during his annual hunting trip—so the fish and wildlife personnel wouldn't mistake him for an endangered species, or one of the grizzly bears, wolves, lions, or even elk that they sometimes put radio collars on in order to justify their employment.

One more anecdote about Jim, now known by everybody as "Shit Coulee": I had just finished replacing a prolapsed uterus on one of Jim's cows. I had hung my down coat on a barbed-wire fence to get it out of the way, but as I released the cow she was a little ill-tempered and charged it. This put a foot-long rip in the fabric, and a stream of goose feathers spewed out into the hills of the Blackfeet Reservation for miles. It was another call when I didn't know whether or not I had broke even financially.

When I went back to the ranch to say good-bye, Shit Coulee invited me in for coffee and told me that he was again having a little trouble with the law. He had come out of his house one morning to see a grizzly bear licking his chops after finishing off a calf Jim had in a pen. Jim ran back in the house to get a gun and his revolver. He jumped into his pickup and caught up to the bear—he told me he shot a few times in her direction in order to scare her so she wouldn't return.

After quite a few of those scare-shots, the bear finally expired, so Jim called the game warden and related the incident to him. The trapper and warden came out and arrested Jim for destroying an animal on the endangered species list, then fined him an enormous amount of money.

Jim asked for a jury trial, and since the Fish and Game Commission and the National Park Service didn't want any veterinarians around their overgrown Boy Scout bureaucracies, they hadn't done a proper necropsy—and Jim was acquitted. No one will ever know for sure what killed that bear, whether it was lead poisoning or the fear of God that Jim had put into him.

THE GAY PIG

ONE MIGHT CALL THIS a "shaggy hog story." But most of it is true.

My friend Jack from Pendroy asked me one night if I would stop by and look at a weird pig of his, which wasn't doing very well. Pendroy was quite a little town in its heyday, consisting of a bank, at least one church, two stores, a post office, three grain elevators, a stockyard with livestock scales, two rural fire departments, one parking meter, and a large real estate and insurance office, administered by the self-appointed Mayor John Swanson. It also had a school and a railroad, being the terminus of a Great Northern Railway spur into a very productive area. In this special little town, Porky was a special pig.

He was the last one born in a litter of eleven piglets. All of his litter mates were white, but he was reddish brown. His dam had only ten teats, so he was able to get very little nourishment—occasionally he sucked a hind teat that one of his siblings had abandoned. He quickly became the runt. Porky's litter mates had all of their canine baby teeth clipped off and their tails removed, as is the custom in pig production, but the odd brown pig missed this operation and ran around with a curly tail and all of his canine teeth intact. He could occasionally fight off the other pigs, but when he finally secured an unused teat on the dam, those sharp little teeth must have traumatized his mother's mammary glands. The sow would roll on her belly and cut him off.

To counteract this tendency, Porky developed a very loud squeal when he was hungry. In order to quiet him Jack's children took pity. They began to treat him as a welfare pig, supplementing his diet three or four times a day with milk replacer. This treatment nearly brought him up to par with his litter mates, but his own pig brothers and sisters began to shun him and fight him if he came near. When the other siblings were weaned from the sow, Porky was returned to the weaning pen with them, but he was ostracized. His bloodcurdling squeals had necessitated his removal from the pens.

Alone, Porky began to take advantage of his circumstance. He had free access to the farm, and learned to penetrate all fences. He was returned to the pigpen—but instead of being shunned, he was now favored. All the rest of the pigs tried to make love to him. This constant attention to his hindquarters caused all his hair to be rubbed off, and he

41

was renamed "Sweet Ass Porky," or the Gay Pig. Because of this condition, Porky was cut back rather than sent to market. He must have felt lonely without the others, since he ran away for two months. Perhaps he tried to find them.

It was when he unexpectedly returned that Jack asked me to take a look at him. We went out together to examine this strange pig, which I noticed immediately had wrinkles. I commented on it, and Jack asked, "What does that mean?"

"It means that he used to be bigger," I said. I also noted that his ears seemed a bit more pointed than the usual pig's, and that he had long, shaggy hair. "He must have been out trying to find himself," I said, "searching for his cultural background." His overall looks reminded me of a genuine Arkansas razorback hog.

"What about his squealing and his sweet-ass tendencies?" Jack inquired.

"Well," I said, "what can you expect from a runty pig that didn't know who his father was, disowned from his brothers and sisters, and neglected by his mother. He's been on welfare his whole life, and squeals whenever you try to take him off his benefits."

"What should I do with him?"

"We'll worm him today, then you should put him in a hog-tight fence with another odd pig," I advised. "That'll keep them in hog heaven until the next batch of pigs are sent to market."

THE TRIP

WE HAD NEVER TAKEN a family vacation. My life as a veterinarian kept us close to home, and neither my wife nor I had any particular desire to wander away from the roots we had established in our pleasant village. We kept busy and occupied, so time slipped by. But at last, in these our golden years, we made the decision to take a trip.

My wife Pat—who I sometimes call Mom, or Grandma, or whatever title fits the occasion—and I decided to make no definite itinerary and make only a general plan of where we were going. We made no reservations and no commitments, except for agreeing to meet a grandson in Los Angeles who misses his native Montana and its fishing, skiing, and mountain pack trips.

What follows is a journal of that once-in-a-lifetime trip:

DAY ONE

We get up at four in the morning after a fitful night of sleep and start the preparations for our great journey. We pack twice the amount of clothing we need, and half the amount of money. Every crack and cranny in our vehicle is stuffed with bags, coats, shoes, flat irons, hair curlers, snow boots, overshoes, blankets, flashlights, boot jacks, shoe horns, swimsuits, coat hangers, wine, and snacks. Since it's January, we even take our skis, poles, and all the paraphernalia that goes with the sport. We want to be prepared for any occasion.

We finally depart at five, and spend the first twenty miles in quiet thought trying to remember what we forgot. Spectacles? Heat turned down? Stove off? Doors locked, windows shut? Happy days! Away we go.

Our first stop is Great Falls, where we drop off some documents at our son's home before proceeding down the great Missouri River to Helena, Montana. The river is steamy in the cold morning. We always enjoy the ride through the spectacular rock formations, but this time we are treated to a beautiful sunrise. We arrive in Helena at seven-thirty, and have to make a brief stop on official business: at a meeting, I learn the lovely Missouri River contains arsenic, and that the state has filed ecological impact statements concerning its water quality. But the pollution is not from mining, or another human source. Instead, the Missouri

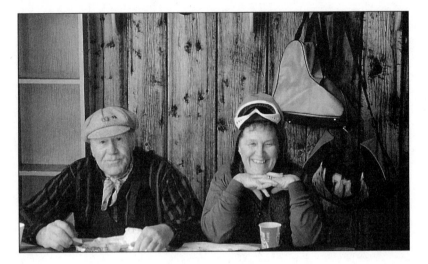

A couple of seniors on a skiing trip.

River's Madison branch originates at Old Faithful geyser in Yellowstone Park and on its course through the park picks up enough minerals from the hot springs and mud pots to exceed EPA tolerances. People who have been drinking this water all their lives are finding out that they should be dead. Oh, well. Maybe next summer the environmentalists will hold a protest march around Old Faithful geyser.

After the meeting, vacation begins in earnest. We spend the rest of the day in the state museum, which displays an artistic— and materialistic—record of Montana's history.

DAY TWO

At dawn, we leave Helena and make a 130-mile sprint to Bozeman and a day of skiing at Big Sky Resort. We dig in every nook and cranny in the car to retrieve our ski clothes, leaving the remainder of our belongings in utter chaos. We soon find out that this will be the rule for the trip: whenever we need something, we find it at the bottom of the pile. Or in the last place we look.

Big Sky ski area was a brainchild of Montana-born news commentator Chet Huntley, who convinced Chrysler Corporation to invest in its development. Economic bailouts and time have removed Chrysler from the scene, but the resort on Lone Mountain is still around and getting bigger every day. It is a good place to enjoy some of Montana's magnificent topography. Following one of the area's newest trails this time, I journeyed over one ridge too many and found myself overlooking a fifty-foot cliff. This separated me from Pat for some time as I inquired of some cross-country *langlaufers* about a course back to a chairlift. A few more cautious runs used up our supply of cholesterol for proper muscle coordination, so we were done recreating for the day.

After parting with one of our sons, who lives in Bozeman and has joined us for the day, we head up the valley for Yellowstone and points south. As we progress up the Gallatin we pass the spot where some bank robbers met their demise after holding up one of Bozeman's institutions in the early 1930s. We observe mountain sheep and elk herds along the river bottoms—and also the stark burned trees from the great Yellowstone forest fires of 1988.

We pass over the divide and into Grayling Creek and the high plateau of Yellowstone. Then we proceed through West Yellowstone, the snowmobile capital of Montana, and drive south over Targhee Pass, between Montana and Idaho. As we head toward the Continental Divide and Pacific watershed, we gape at the beautiful, snow-covered terrain! We natives tend to take things for granted.

We stay the night in Driggs, Idaho, and tomorrow will make another day of skiing—this time at Grand Targhee, on the west side of the Grand Tetons.

DAY THREE

At Targhee, we have always found the skiing superb and deep powder galore. Ten inches of new snow greet us when we wake. We cover the mountains more like frivolous teenagers than like senior citizens. Skiing through untracked powder for four to five hours uses up calories, and after we're done for the day we find a delightful restaurant with a professional New York chef to meet our needs. If the fur trappers who attended the rendezvous in Pierre's Hole in 1834 could have dined as elegantly as we did, they would have forgotten all about the pelting business and carved a few ski runs. What a place!

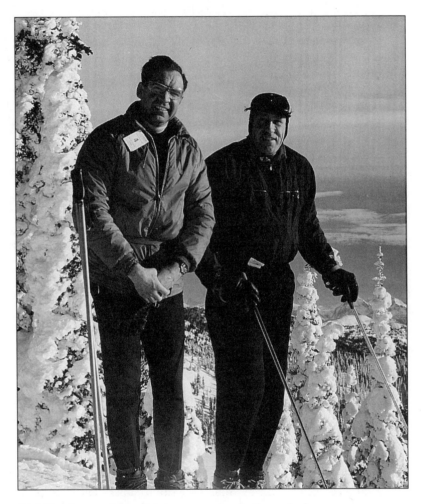

Dick Voorhees and another top competitor in the early days.

DAY FOUR

Out to the interstate. We drive through immense grain and potato fields blanketed with snow, across creeks and rivers, over deep lava cliffs and rocky canyons, and onto high mesas and mountainous divides. We flow with the traffic, proceeding across the former Oregon Trail and

Idaho's immense lava beds. We wind our way down to the Great Salt Lake and bed down for the night near the spot where the rails of the first intercontinental railroad were joined with a golden spike.

DAY FIVE

The Great Salt Lake holds more water than it has for years and nearly laps at the banks of the highway. Nestled between two great mountain ranges, it is a sight to see as we go by. Since we were not yet burned out from skiing, we skirt Salt Lake City, capital of the Latter-Day Saints, and head up Little Cottonwood Canyon to the old mining site of Alta in the Wasatch Mountains. Alta has eighteen to twenty inches of new snow. After its staff drops a few hand grenades from a helicopter to ward off avalanches, and after another hour detainment we termed "interlock," we head up the mountain to the greatest powder skiing in the world.

When I first went skiing at Alta, the area had no paved roads, one chairlift, and one permanent resident—Mayor Watson, who was left over from the mining days. A group of winter sports advocates including Joe Quinny began the development. The resort's manager today is Onno Weiringa III, a local man from our hometown of Conrad. It now has at least ten chairlifts, many accommodations, and, best of all, the best and most consistent snow conditions in the world. Nearby is family, of sorts— Stanley Steamer, one of the best quarter horses I ever raised, who is now owned by Onno.

Cowboy, skier, avalanche expert, resort manager, river rafter Onno and his wife put us up for the night, and Pat and I enjoy some of the best powder skiing of our lives. We had spent our last vacation there together in 1953—we were on our honeymoon. The skiing was good then, but it's even better today.

DAY SIX

We ski until we "burn out," then head south to continue our trip. On the busy highway, every other vehicle is a sixteen- or eighteen-wheeler, many with pups or trailers behind. Either trains aren't hauling much American merchandise anymore, or the trucking industry is doing a superfine job. We pass by orchards, irrigated land, and Mormon churches in a land that nearly fulfills Brigham Young's dream of the promised land.

THE TRIP

We pass the great mines and smelters at Provo next. A few miles farther on, we leave the busy interstate highway and head southwest to cross a mountain range and drop down to the coal mines of Price, Utah. Here they ship the coal out and slurry it out by pipeline. Such a slurry pipe is controversial because it takes many, many gallons of precious liquid away from an arid country. And when I say arid, I mean it. This desert makes my armpits look like wetlands. The Green River, as we cross it, appears to be only ankle-deep. The Colorado River at the city of Moab couldn't float a duck, let alone a raft.

When we get to Price, the museum is closed and the pawn shop is busy. Since the weather was nice and warm compared to what we know in Montana, we continue on our way south ahead of an impending storm forecast by the media sages.

The increased altitude of the Four Corners country—at the intersection of Utah, Colorado, New Mexico, and Arizona—opens a new panorama. Farms, ranches, and livestock appear. Coyotes dart across the highways and the grain fields remind me of home. Cortez, Colorado, could be transplanted to Montana and fit in with places like Plains, Hot Springs, and Paradise.

With a full tank of gas to put our mind at ease, my good navigator and I speed on ahead of the pending weather to new country and more titillation. Soon we are awarded the grand sight of volcanic Ship Rock in New Mexico. It's spectacular at sunset, and the last rays of sunshine bring out the outlines and shadows and thrill both Pat and me. We promise ourselves to spend more time here the next go-round.

We drive down the San Juan Valley and eventually succumb to the travelers' "rump-sprung" feeling and darkness. Farmington, New Mexico, is our stopover, where we have a hasty steak in a supper club/bar filled with oil workers disguised as cowboys, or cowboys turned roustabouts. Beer, hats, tight jeans, a loud jukebox, and a stoic Native American couple provide us with our topics of conversation.

DAY SEVEN

The big snowstorm hits as we pull out of Farmington the next morning on our way to Santa Fe. Curving mountain roads and poor visibility limit our view. I hold on to the steering wheel while Pat does most of the

48

navigating. Rigor mortis sets in and complaints of nausea from vertigo are heard as we pass through the blizzard and around trucks spewing rooster-tails of snow a quarter of a mile behind them. When the traffic is light, we turn on the radio and hear reports of ninety-seven-mile-an-hour winds in Albuquerque. Just like home.

We shortcut over the Continental Divide again, through the Abiquiu country where artist Georgia O'Keeffe lived, and into the valley of the Rio Grande. As we close in on Santa Fe and the world of Spanish names, customs, and people, we find its inhabitants are happy for the moisture brought by the storm. It takes two to three inches of water per day in this climate to keep plants growing. An old cottonwood tree will transpire around five hundred gallons of water per day.

We find a motel in the center of the city and start a pedestrian tour of Santa Fe's galleries, jewelry shops, and all of the varied and many things New Mexico's state capital provides.

DAYS EIGHT AND NINE

On to San Diego and the Pacific Ocean. After a long drive across a dry land, we visit our relatives in a beautiful ocean-front condominium overlooking a wide, white beach on the vast Pacific. What a relaxing change for a couple of Montana natives! We can't believe there are strollers, beachcombers, surfers, swimmers enjoying the summerlike climate—of January! We join the strollers and watch huge naval aircraft carriers coming and going. It brings back the memories and days I spent as a naval aviator during World War II. Like the call of the wild, the call of the sea and ports unknown still evoke profound yearnings in me.

DAY TEN

Talk about people's yearnings. California is one vast example of those. We leave San Diego and crawl to Los Angeles in a maze of vehicles and traffic that makes us yearn, in turn, for the isolation of our own Montana.

An old saying goes, "The good Lord passed out brains on a square-mile basis." California's too cramped to give anyone much room to think. California drivers are proof of this. I'm certain some of them have the same opinion of my abilities that I have of theirs. I know this because they did not hesitate to tell me so in both verbal and sign language.

We finally arrive in the "city of angels" and pick up our grandson.

DAYS ELEVEN AND TWELVE

These are the highlight of the trip. Our grandson Connor is in California living with his mother after a divorce. After we pick him out of a kindergarten that looks more like a prison than a school, we spend time spoiling him and catering to all his wishes. We stay with our youngest son and his beautiful wife, observing the ways of life and the moves of people crowded together in this imitation of the Garden of Eden.

But somehow, it all falls flat. I guess I would rather be cold and alone than squeezed into a can like a sardine and sprayed for fruit flies amid the smog of diesel smoke and industry.

DAY THIRTEEN

Leaving L.A. and its incoming traffic on a Monday morning makes me thankful I don't have my humor challenged like this on a daily basis. We take the fastest route out of the Golden State into the wastelands of the Nevada desert, where we can at last breathe a sigh of relief as the traffic disappears. Once again we can watch the scenery in tranquillity.

Pat takes over the driving chores and we arrive in Winnemucca for an evening of gaming and gambling. We can do the same thing in Montana, but it's more fun and sporty a thousand miles from home. The outcome is the same, however—our pocketbooks are considerably lighter as we pack up the next morning to continue the trip.

DAY FOURTEEN

We drive into the center of a big snowstorm in southeastern Oregon and spend the next few hours counting the mishaps of fellow travelers unused to winter conditions. Truck traffic ceases in the whiteout. Truckers are pulled off at truck stops or at the bottoms of long grades, putting on chains. I don't envy them their profession. We have our hands full herding one little auto between the two ditches, but with my wife's sage advice and help, we make it past the worst parts.

After a hard go, we drop into the valley of Snake River and find roads that once again are bare and dry. We stop for lunch and a visit with an

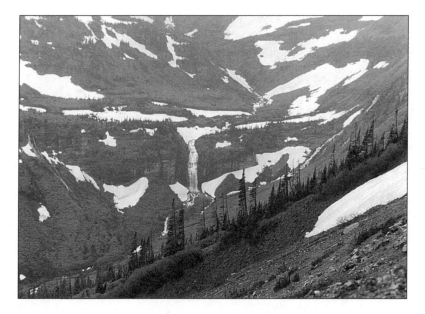

Cold but gorgeous country in Glacier National Park.

old friend from my student days at Colorado A & M University. He is up on me by a couple of marriages and seven kids, but he's still in active practice as a veterinarian. With all his wives and children he probably can't afford to retire.

We then continue our journey north through snow country, mountains, and icy roads to LaGrande, Oregon, where we spend the evening curing the evils of the world. My friend Hugh McNamer, a gifted Irish real-estate man, shows me a video on a big ranch hereabouts that raises Limousin cattle. But I decided that one ranch is enough for me—our holdings on the Two Medicine River in Montana will take care of our needs and investments for the rest of our lives.

DAY FIFTEEN

After partaking a most delicious breakfast that probably adds two more pounds to the extra ones I've already collected from this new life of travel and leisure, Pat and I take off on the final leg of our journey. We pass Pendleton, Oregon; Spokane, Washington; Coeur d'Alene, Idaho;

THE TRIP

Lookout Pass (with two feet of new snow and still snowing); Missoula, Montana; and the Continental Divide again, at Rogers Pass.

Just as we get lonesome for our own house and bed, we notice that one little difference has occurred: the car windows have begun to frost. As we drop off the Rocky Mountain Front onto the prairie where we live, I punch the exterior temperature gauge. It sends me a reading of twenty-six degrees below zero, and I know we are getting close to home sweet home.

It's no wonder that we folks in the Big Sky Country live in isolation. It's damn cold outside.

WIND BELLY

HOLLOW BELLY IS THE CONDITION of not getting enough to eat. Compare that to wind belly, which is getting too much to eat—but too much of food with such low nutritional value that an animal has to eat enormous amounts in order to survive. In my years of veterinary practice, I've seen many instances of both of these varieties of essentially the same disease—starvation.

One cold morning when the temperature was about thirty degrees below zero, my friend Harold called me. "Are you busy this morning?" he asked.

"Yes," I said, as I sat next to the warm stove toasting my toes after a brief exposure to the morning weather. It was bitter out there, with a wind-chill factor of about fifty-below. I very seldom wore a face mask, but I'd need one that day. I could tell by the sting on my face that my cheeks were not going to survive prolonged exposure to the cold north wind and driving snow that had put icicles on my eyebrows and eyelashes.

It wasn't just the cold—I really did have plans. I was inspecting a herd of cattle that I had treated the previous day for coccidiosis, an intestinal parasite that eats away the lining of the gut and results in hemorrhagic diarrhea. It was either too cold for the cattle to defecate, or the medicine was very effective.

It was as I stepped out of the car to close the gate that the wind and the cold hit me briefly. Suddenly satisfied that the treatment and my efforts had improved the herd's health, I decided to head back to the animal hospital. I turned the heater on full-blast to thaw out a little as I drove, and hoped that no one else would call. I thought I could catch up on indoor work, like small-animal surgery or book work for my friends in the Internal Revenue Service.

But Harold's call had disturbed me. He was tighter than the rectal sphincter muscle on a day when one is afflicted simultaneously with flatulence and diarrhea. (That reminds me of a cowboy friend of mine who thought diarrhea was hereditary because it ran in your jeans.) "Oh, well," I sighed. The business of veterinary medicine in Northern Montana is no job for a sissy, and I knew that Harold was in trouble. He wouldn't give me the honor of treating his animals if he could do it himself.

As I reluctantly turned the warming car toward his place, I felt a stinging sensation in one earlobe. When I reached up to feel it, it was frozen solid as an ice cube. I wondered if I might lose the thing, and have to grow long hair and go through the rest of my life like Vincent Van Gogh. But it was a quick freeze job, and resulted only in a future sensitivity to cold weather.

When I reached his place, Harold told me that he was losing cattle. The weather had been cold for an extended period and, although a frugal man, he had thrown out copious amounts of straw for them to eat and bed down on. On my arrival at his ranch, I reached a diagnosis of wind belly. The cows had eaten so much straw and drunk so little water that most of the "Golden Oldies," "Short Termers," or "Plum Gums," as I often called older animals because their teeth had all fallen out, were suffering from compaction of the rumen, one of the four compartments of the stomach.

There are mainly two treatments for this condition, neither very successful under stress conditions. One is the surgical removal of the compacted mass, and the other is pumping of at least one gallon of mineral oil into the rumen, plus a cathartic agent to stimulate gut movement. I could speak to the effectiveness of mineral oil myself—I can recall taking a tablespoon of the stuff, administered by my mother, for a constipation complaint. The resulting effusion of intestinal contents ended forever my complaints of stomachaches. From then on, I answered the inevitable question, "Have you gone to the bathroom lately or had a bowel movement?" in the positive.

Back to Harold's herd. In spite of the day being very cold, I removed the compaction from two of the cows by surgery. I also treated two others with mineral oil. In order to use the supply I had carried with me, I had to heat it. When it's twenty degrees below zero, mineral oil is like Vaseline, which, after all, is essentially the same stuff. I dosed the cows, and before I left told Harold he had better get another fifty-five gallon drum of mineral oil and be prepared for the worst.

I called him the next day and learned that my surgical survival rate was fifty percent. The mineral oil treatment hadn't shown outstanding results, but it seemed to have broken down the compactions. One cow was showing some diarrhea. All of the afflicted animals were still eat-

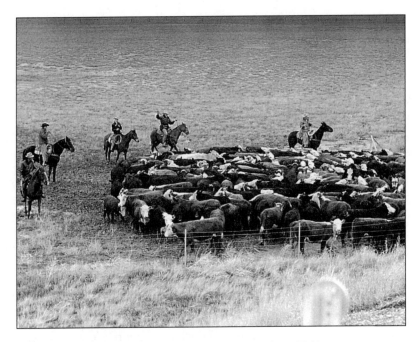

Driving five hundred head to the Shelby Stockyards in 1963.

ing—and Harold was following my nutritional advice, which was to change the herd's diet to a good-quality hay and a high-energy cake or cubed ground cereal. Harold had also purchased the drum of mineral oil. After a little more conversation, and after he'd inquired about my fee, he decided that my services were no longer needed.

Cattle prices were not very good at the time, and even though I'd put in cold weather duty Harold never did pay me in cash. I ended up trading my fee for his training of a racehorse—which I also had traded for. About that time I realized that financial gains were not easy to come by in this region. It was just as easy to go backwards and lose your ass as it was to go forward and freeze it.

WINTER UNDERWEAR

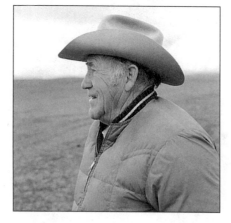

Staying warm in the field.

MY FRIEND GEORGE always wanted to be a brand inspector. He had a few feathers in his hat, and his connection with the Blackfeet Tribe finally landed him a job with the Montana Livestock Commission. He was named assistant brand inspector at the stockyards where I inspected cattle for health at weekly sales.

Not long after George got the job, during one of the big fall runs, a northern blizzard moved in and drove the wind-chill factor down to about sixty degrees below zero. I believe it was the Captains Lewis and Clark who mentioned the fact that one of the several people they treated during their first winter in our northern climate had "frozen his dally whacker." I know from personal experience that genital organs tend to shrink and nearly disappear into the body cavities when exposed to such severe weather, especially if one is only wearing a pair of chaps and astride a horse when one of our cold spells hits. Your legs, feet, and other anatomical parts turn purple, and it doesn't take long to develop frostbite and hypothermia.

George had not prepared himself for the ravages of such a cold snap. After several hours of being miserable as he checked cattle brands, he asked his superior if he could go home and put on his long underwear and find some warmer winter clothing. He was given permission and left.

George never showed up again that afternoon. About twenty-four hours later, he called and said he would be back to work as soon as he could.

"Where are you?" his boss asked.

"In Browning," he replied.

"I thought you just went home to put on your long underwear!"

"I did," said George. "I just forgot to tell you it was up here in Browning"—two hundred miles away.

RASPUTIN

I CAN'T THINK OF MANY veterinarians who have not had a patient run away, hide, or escape completely from their premises. Although we take precautions and warn all employees that it is not only embarrassing, but negligent—since the hospitalization of a patient puts the responsibility for its care under our jurisdiction—breakaways still happen. You've read already that animals are not dumb. They must plot against us to get revenge for the shots and uncomfortable treatments that are required for their health.

Cats are probably the worst, because they become scared more easily around strangers and can hide much more easily. They can secrete themselves right under your eyes and remain hidden for days until hunger and thirst finally drive them out of seclusion, allowing for their capture. Cats seldom, if ever, respond to commands as dogs do, since they're too independent and adverse to training. They also are expert climbers and have been known to climb curtains, walls, poles, trees, or anything that is vertical. Don't be fooled—this goes for declawed pets as well.

When blue-pointed Siamese cats were still rare, in the early days of my practice, everyone seemed to want one. One day a lady came in with a beautiful Siamese and politely asked if I could find a nice home for it. She told me that it was a curtain climber and had ruined enough curtains to bankrupt her. It seemed to want to look down on everyone, and thought of its domicile as the top of a frilly curtain rod. If its owner happened to forget that the cat was there and opened or closed the curtain, the cat would take a startling leap and "scare the hell out of anything or anyone around," she said.

I had no trouble in finding that faddish creature a new home. In fact, I found five new homes for that one cat, and I didn't make many friends in the process. The Siamese never got over its ability to destroy curtains and rods. A house cat, it could sneak into its new owner's living room, or wherever she or he didn't want it, practically unnoticed. It had other flaws, too. It wasn't very neat in its bowel movement habits and could spread kitty litter record distances. And its appetite was voracious, which only made changing the kitty litter harder and required such change more often.

RASPUTIN

After two or three owners had returned the fashionable beast to me, I secretly wished it was a runaway cat and could consequently "get lost." I even thought of paying a ransom to get someone else to guarantee it a suitable home. I'd pay well, if they'd only promise never to return it.

In between its numerous adoption trials, the cat had full run of the hospital. Since it had been pampered from the time it was a small kitten, it was always in the way. A feline that has had its tail stepped on is a mind-boggling experience. If you accidentally step on a cat, you might as well just throw everything in the air and run. Otherwise, you'll collapse from the shock of the cat's response—or else just get the hell scared out of you. You'll remain that way for at least a day or two until the memory gradually fades. The cat that was so often underfoot became quite well known around the hospital, and I gave it the evil name of Rasputin.

Just about the time I was getting used to him, the hospital crew decided that Rasputin must go. They took out an advertisement on the local radio "pet parade" and in the local newspaper, and finally found a home with a lonesome old cowboy friend of mine. The match was perfect—the cowboy's shack had no curtains. He didn't mind the cat tipping over the Sego condensed milk can every now and then, and after years of listening to mountain lions screeching through the night he wasn't too startled when Rasputin gave the trampled tail appendage yell. The old gent considered Rasputin a good mouser and they became fast friends until age took its toll and the cat disappeared.

I can still recall one image of their long-lasting relationship. One morning I looked out and saw the cowboy starting out on a morning horseback ride. His favorite dog trotted out in front of the horse he was riding, and Rasputin followed along behind. That cat had his tail in the air and was strutting, displaying his natural beauty to the entire world.

THE NEIGHBOR'S WIFE

THIS BIT OF MEMORABILIA doesn't particularly relate to the practice of veterinary medicine. It relates more to my neighbor and the friendships developed by sharing and caring during the early days of my practice in a small town in Montana.

When my wife and I were first married, we rented a house in a new development that was aptly nicknamed Diaperville. The prolific creation of progeny in this era after World War II was phenomenal in all of the look-alike houses.

The exception to the otherwise parental neighbors was the couple who lived next door, Ade and Dorothy. Ade was an easygoing, wine-drinking bricklayer. Dorothy was a gregarious hypochondriac with a heart problem that she claimed precluded reproduction. This was the reason they had made no addition to posterity or the neighborhood.

These neighbors did, however, have a cat, which I usually took care of. They were also grateful to me for having removed a skunk from their back porch after Ade had shot it—the noise and odor woke everyone in the relatively peaceful neighborhood that night, and lights were on in every house in the vicinity. As an animal-based professional, I was appointed to remove the source of the odoriferous scent. After I put the dead skunk in an airtight garbage sack, I gave Ade orders to scrub the porch out with ammonia and tomato juice and left a variety of odor-masking sprays to make their house and vicinity livable. For the next week it was not difficult to find a conversational topic over any backyard fence.

I came home to our cookie-cutter house one evening to find my yard well manicured. Ade had returned my skunk favor with gratitude, and over a few sips of his wine we struck a deal. If he would mow my lawn in summer, I would shovel his snow in winter. Summer was always a busy time for me, and I relished cleaning sidewalks on frosty winter mornings after a beautiful snowstorm better than chasing a lawnmower around on a hot summer day. I told Ade that I would much rather rope calves or train horses when the weather was nice. Neither one of us conveyed the information of our bargain to our spouses.

The first big snowstorm in November of that year found me out scooping snow off the sidewalks and porches as the sun came up. The sparkling crystals in the atmosphere, the big blue skies, and the snow-clad

THE NEIGHBOR'S WIFE

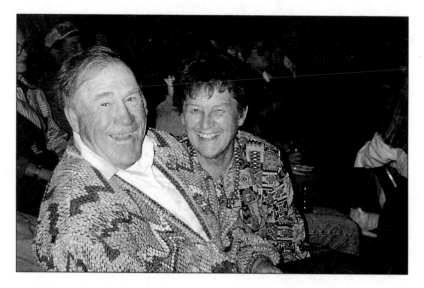

Pat and me just having a little fun.

mountains made my work enjoyable. I first cleared all our walks and approaches, then moved onto Dorothy and Ade's property.

I was putting the finishing touches on their snow removal when Dorothy popped out of her front door and surveyed the situation. She was ever so grateful, she said. She told me she had been nagging Ade for years to get their snow shoveled off quickly. "He's still in bed," she said, adding that he would be very surprised and thankful also.

I knew when she asked me how much she owed me that she had never been informed of our bargain. I thought for a moment before answering her. "Dorothy," I said, "you don't owe me a thing."

"I do," she said. "How much do other folks around here usually pay you?"

"Well," I paused for effect. "That nice lady next door lets me sleep with her."

Dorothy ran back into her house and slammed the door. Never again did she attempt to pay me for shoveling their sidewalks! Come to think of it, I never heard any more about her heart problems, either, and my thought on the subject is that she will probably outlive all of us.

ROOM TO ROAM

AS A VETERINARIAN IN NORTHERN Montana, I have always had room to roam. When I arrived here along the forty-ninth parallel of latitude, I was the only veterinarian in the area. For several years, I logged nearly 100,000 miles per annum, wearing out a car every twelve months. I often pitied the man who was unlucky enough to purchase one of my used-up vehicles, which had been herded between the ditches over gumbo and graveled roads, with holes punched in gas tanks from flying gravel, pitted windows from sand storms and flying rocks, and radiators plugged with insects and misfortunate birds. One year, shortly after I had traded in one of these used cars, the honest car salesman called me over to tell me that the car's new purchaser had asked how long he had to drive it at a reduced speed before it was "broken in," as he put it.

Today, Montana's speed limit is whatever is "reasonable and prudent." For a man in a hurry, what's reasonable is not exactly definitive—it's reasonable that I should drive faster when I'm behind schedule or on an errand of animal mercy. I have never been in an accident, but I've had a few close calls.

My children all learned to drive sitting on instrument cases or pillows, long before they were eligible for drivers' training. By the time they were of proper age, most of them were well-seasoned skinners and seldom pestered me about driving. Once in a while there would be a catastrophe—such as the time my son Erik lost a wheel and petitioned me to write him an excuse for being tardy at school.

When the children grew up and left home for college, they inherited my used cars. One day my sister borrowed one of their cars for a political rally, and the steering wheel came off in her hands. I don't think she ever asked to use one of their cars again.

One of the hazards of country and prairie driving is the loss of mufflers. Today the Midas muffler man usually sticks to his guarantee, but in years gone by there were no muffler shops. I have wired my fair share of mufflers and pipes up with baling wire and barbed wire.

One day, in a snowstorm, I wiped the front wheel off when I didn't hit a cattle guard square. This resulted in a seven-mile hike. Another time I was tootling along on an isolated trail, having a little fun smashing through snowbanks, when—whoops!—I ended up stuck in one of my

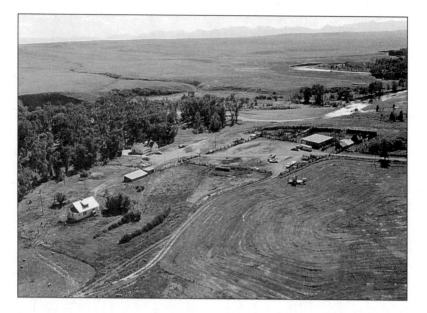

Lots of room at the Cross Three Ranch—and a river runs through it.

targets. I had to dig the car out with my stainless steel veterinary bucket.

I complain a lot, but at heart I cherish the lonesome roads and room to roam. There are only about 1.7 people per square mile in Montana, and most of these live in the state's twelve largest cities. Even though our winters are milder than most, rumors have spread that we live in the coldest spot in the nation. Now every time my wife and I go on one of our infrequent trips and get squeezed in by semi-rigs whose wheels are as high as the top of my car, we start looking for alternative routes that will take us on back roads and deserted highways. How good it is to have a little space around us! We are fortunate to have spent our life in the spacious Big Sky Country, where we can start a log fire and sit next to it in a quiet winter, watching birds, livestock, dogs, and memories go by.

Some Favorite Lyrics and Pertinent Poems

OLD STRAWBERRY'S CASTRATION

Hanging 'round town spending my time,
Out of a job, not earning a dime,
Up steps a fellow and he says, "I suppose
That you're a bronc buster by the looks of your clothes."
"You're guessin' me right and a good one," I claim.
I ask if he's got any tough ones to tame.
He says he's got one that's a good one to buck—
At throwing good riders he's had lots of luck.
He says, "Get your saddle and I'll give you a chance."
We got in the buckboard and drove to the ranch.
There in the corral standing alone,
Stood a ball-bearing stud, a strawberry roan.
I got my loop on him; it sure was a fight.
I threw on my saddle. I screws her down tight.
Then I jump on him and jerk off the blind.
I'm right in his middle. Now watch him unwind.
He hides his old head and I'll say he unwound.
He seemed to quit living down there on the ground.
He goes up in the east and comes down in the west
While I'm in the middle a-doin' my best.
He's the worst buckin' bronc I've seen on the range.
He can turn on a nickel and give you back change.
I first lose a stirrup and then lose my hat.
I start pulling leather, as blind as a bat.
Then old roany, he goes up on high
And leaves me a sittin' way up in the sky.
I turn over twice and come back to earth.
I lay there a-cussin' the day of his birth.
Now the boss steps up and says, "That's enough.
The Old Strawberry stud is too damn tough.
I'm tired of seeing cowboys take falls.
We're going to rope him and carve out his balls."
So I build a big loop and go to the corral.
I snared his front feet as he farted and fell.

The boss jumps on him and holds up his head.
The wind has left him and he acts half-dead.
I tie his old legs, pull out the scalpel.
Then carve his bag as he lets out a big yell.
He squeals like a pig, he shivers and jerks,
And fights like the devil with mouth full of dirt.
All I can find is one of his nuts.
So I rolls my sleeves and dives in his guts.
I thought I had found one when I felt something pass,
But it was only a turd on the way to his ass.
Then I hear a loud scream and thundering squalls
and find out that old Roany has the boss by the balls.
I stomped on his head, but it was of no use.
Just like a pit bull he wouldn't turn loose.
So I untied his legs and he got to his feet.
But the boss's voice changed, and I knew he was beat.
I'll advise you to leave old Roany alone,
He's an ole high-flanker with high testosterone.
But the boss is worse off as you can easily tell,
With no gonads at all, only a high-octave yell.

THE FIRST JOKE I CAN REMEMBER
OR, D.O.A.

The big, fat cat was taking a nap
with its tail over the highway rail.
In its profound sleep it did not hear the beep
and, therefore, lost its tail.
In great surprise it turned around
to see who'd done the ghastly deed.
And before he knew it...he blew it,
for his head followed his tail's lead.

There's a simple moral to this gory story:
Don't lose your head over a piece of tail.

THE OLD WOODSTOVE

When old Cold-Maker spews down from the north
With nothing but fenceposts to alter his course
It's then that I tarry and begin to procrastinate
Even though the kine are gathering at the gate.
I stoke the old stove with an extra log
And take another look at the snow and ground fog.
I turn my back to the pleasant heat
To warm my heart and toast my feet.
The old wood stove feels mighty good
As I stand there listening to the crackling wood.
In a minute or two I'll have to face the weather
But right now I'll take the fire over that refrigerator.

RIB'S SHORT POEM

Uncle George and Auntie Mable
Fainted at the breakfast table.
This should be sufficient warning:
Never do it in the morning.

GEORGE AND MABLE, REVIVED

Oats and bran have set them right.
Now they do it every night.
And Uncle George is hoping soon
That he can do it in the afternoon.

DRINK

When I was young, I drank a beer.
I didn't like the taste,
So I switched to whiskey.
This was risky:
I drank to feel frisky.
Then I drank to sober up and
I drank when I was depressed.
I drank to impress.
I drank till I couldn't remember.
It affected every family member.
To tell you the truth, now that I've quit,
Abstinence doesn't bother me a bit.

Try it, you might like it.

ON AGE

The years slip by faster than you think.
Your eyes grow dim, you lose your hair
And you can't trust your sphincters
When you pass some air!

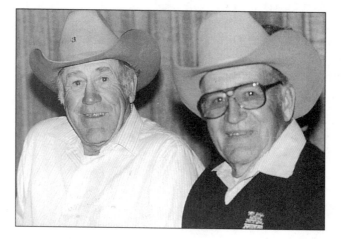

Two cowboy brothers.

THE LITTLE RED HEN

Said the little red hen to the little red rooster,
"You don't come around, sir, as often as you useter."
Said the little red rooster to the little red hen,
"I'll meet you in the barnyard about half past ten."

Oh the night was dark and you could hardly see,
The little red hen cried out with glee.
Said the little red hen to the little red rooster,
"You are much better, sir, than you ever useter."

Said a big gruff voice,
"This ain't no rooster."
It was then that the little red hen knew
The gander had goosed her!

CHANGING THE ENVIRONMENT

The other day I slipped and fell.
When I looked around I found the cause:
Twas a very fresh cow pie.
I cursed the environment.
Today as I look at the snowcapped mountains,
The greening hills, and the crystal-clear water,
The grazing cattle and cavorting deer,
A thought came back and I changed my mind.
I love my environment.

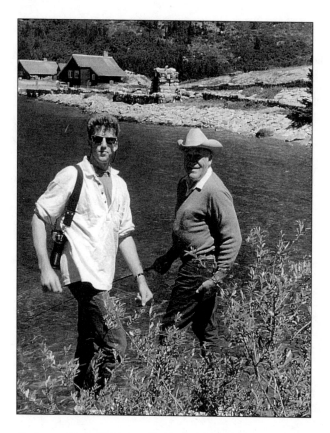

Father and son fishing at Swift Current.

ONE LAST TOAST

I've drunk to your health on the range
I've toasted your health at home
I drank to your health so often
I damn near ruined my own.